# THE
# SUPER*foods*
# DIET BOOK

Also by Michael Van Straten and Barbara Griggs,
published by Dorling Kindersley
**SUPERFOODS**

# THE
# SUPER*foods*
# DIET BOOK

MICHAEL VAN STRATEN
AND
BARBARA GRIGGS

**DORLING KINDERSLEY**
LONDON · NEW YORK · STUTTGART

A DORLING KINDERSLEY BOOK

**Project Editor:** Jane Mason
**Designer:** Peter Laws
**Managing Editor:** Krystyna Mayer
**Managing Art Editor:** Derek Coombes
**Production Manager:** Maryann Rogers
Illustrations by Madeleine David

First published in Great Britain in 1992
by Dorling Kindersley Limited
9 Henrietta Street, London WC2E 8PS

**Visit us on the World Wide Web at**
http://www.dk.com

Reprinted 1992, 1993 (twice), 1994 (twice), 1996

A CIP catalogue record for this book is available from The British Library

ISBN 0-86318-749-8

**A Jill Norman Book**

Typeset by Dorchester Typesetting Group Limited, Dorcheser, UK
Printed and bound in Singapore by Star Standard Industries (PTE) Ltd.

# CONTENTS

## ACKNOWLEDGMENTS

The authors would like to thank the following authors and publishers
for permission to quote recipes from their work:
Janet Ross and Michael Waterfield: *Leaves from our Tuscan Kitchen*,
(John Murray)
Arto der Haroutunian: *Classic Vegetable Cookery*, (Thorsons)
Colin Spencer: *Cordon Vert*, (Thorsons)
John Edwards: *The Roman Cookery of Apicius*, (Rider)
Philippa Davenport: *Country Living Country Cook*, (Ebury Press)
Elizabeth David: *Spices, Salt and Aromatics in the English Kitchen*,
(Penguin) and *A Book of Mediterranean Food* (Dorling Kindersley).
They would also like to thank Lynn Bartlett, catering manager at
Waddesdon Manor for the National Trust, who created many of the
delicious recipes in this book; Margery Brooks, who tested a number
of recipes for us; the Fresh Fruit and Vegetable Bureau, and the
Scottish Salmon Information Service for other recipes.

# MESSAGE FROM THE AUTHORS

*B*etween us, we have had decades of involvement with health and nutrition. We have dealt with the practical problems of patients, readers, and listeners. We've delved into research from all over the world. We've looked at every diet fad – and tried out some of them ourselves. And we've examined all the extreme health regimes, ranging from the religious privations of the East to the lunatic excesses of Hollywood. So what follows in this book is, we are certain, the only sensible, practical, enjoyable and, above all, healthy way to achieve and maintain the weight that Nature intended for you.

The Superfoods way of eating is simple, safe, and effective. You certainly don't need to consult a doctor before you follow this plan. If all you want to do is to lose some weight, just turn to p.30, master the simple rules, and follow the Superfoods Diet, with the help of our delicious recipes and menus.

However, we would urge you to read the other chapters. Not only will they help you understand why the Superfoods Diet works. They will also explain why all those boring, difficult, antisocial diets of deprivation were such disastrous failures. If any one of them had worked, you wouldn't be reading this book.

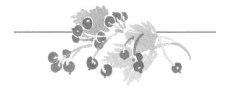

# INTRODUCTION

*On those who prescribe diets: if they do no other*
*good, they prepare their patients betimes for death,*
*by gradually undermining and cutting off*
*their enjoyment of life*
(MICHEL DE MONTAIGNE, 1595)

We hesitated at first to call this the Superfoods Diet; even four centuries ago, the word had acquired a meaning virtually the opposite of its original significance. It's the same today. Most people understand "diet" as an unpleasant regime of severe food restriction which one "goes on" in order to lose weight. What Diet originally meant, and still does in its proper context, is the routine, regular daily intake of food: in other words, eating. There is only one constituent of a good diet: good food.

The Superfoods Diet is exactly what it says: a regular, routine pattern of eating, which is healthy, pleasant, and extremely easy to follow. The bonus of the Superfoods Diet is that you will lose weight if you need to. You think you've got a weight problem? You've probably got half a dozen diet books on your shelf already. Now you can throw them all away – you just need enough room for this one!

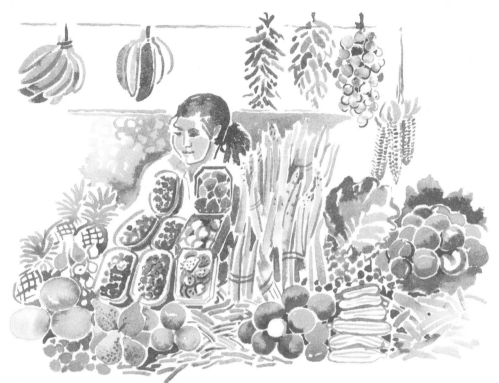

Read this book – and you'll never need to diet again. Dieting doesn't work. The Superfoods Diet does. The philosophy of this book is to banish from your life forever the guilt, the misery, the obsession, and the sense of failure you may have lived with for years as you struggled with one dreary and impossible diet after another.

Eating should be enjoyable – whether it's a simple omelette and salad on your own, a packed lunch at your desk in the office, a hearty Sunday lunch with the family, or sitting around a table with good friends, good food, and a glass of good wine. Eating is one of life's great pleasures, and anything which deprives you of that pleasure, or makes you feel guilty about enjoying what you eat can only be harmful.

Whether you want to lose a few pounds – or a few stone – the Superfoods Diet will do it for you. You need never go on a "diet" again. You need never feel hungry or deprived. You need never turn down another invitation for fear of "sinning". You will be the weight you want to be if you master the simple principles of the Superfoods Diet.

**Good food
makes a
good diet**

CHAPTER 1

# WHO SAYS YOU SHOULD LOSE WEIGHT?

Dieting is the number one obsession of our age. How many people do you know who never talk about dieting? You can probably count them on the fingers of one hand. How many dieters, though, are actually overweight enough to warrant the miseries they inflict on themselves, and those around them, in their endless quest for thinness? This modern obsession has two roots: one of them is the epidemic of obesity – a direct result of the world-wide, multi-billion-dollar food industry, which pours out a cornucopia of high-fat, high-sugar, refined, processed, and denatured food. While millions starve in the under-developed countries, other millions in the affluent West suffer from a twentieth-century disease – overconsump-tion malnutrition, a condition where the body may be deprived of vital nutrients while awash with empty calories. Obesity, the conse-quence of overconsumption, is endemic in the West today. When the Yankee stadium is full, 12,000 of the 100,000 spectators will be grotesquely overweight. There are 20,000,000 excessively fat citizens of the United States – the world's richest country. Even in stylish Italy, where *bella figura* is a national obsession, five in every 100 adults are severely overweight. When the Pope addresses the faithful in St. Peter's Square, he looks down on 5,000 obese worshippers in the crowd of 100,000.

The other – psychological – cause of today's obsession with weight problems is relentless pressure from the media, the fashion dictators, the entertainment business, and the slimming industry itself. All of them send out the same message: Thin is In and Stout is Out. Serious

**Dieting is the great obsession of our age**

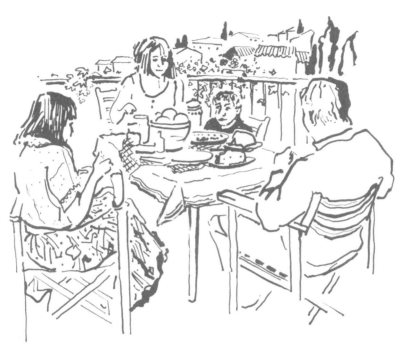

obesity is undoubtedly a real health hazard. But unnecessary dieting and the obsession with weight-loss may pose a more serious risk to our health – physical as well as mental – than a few surplus pounds.

## MEDIA MANIPULATION

The modern thinness cult isn't even a century old. In Queen Victoria's time, or the expansive Edwardian age, the great beauties of the day were often ample, voluptuous, and splendidly curved. A stroll around any art gallery will show you the generous splendours of Rubens's or Rembrandt's women. The Venus de Milo must have been at least a size 18. Most of the women painted by Renoir would be firmly directed to the Outsize Department in any department store today.

The rot set in during the 1920s. Flappers were all the rage and their clothes looked best on skinny bodies. For years the Duchess of Windsor headed the Best-dressed List. Her motto was "You can never be too thin or too rich". Biba and Mary Quant were the fashion names that made news in the 1960s. The mini wasn't made for Juno, and their ranges started at size 6. "Dolly-birds" were by definition tiny. All the fashion designers seem to have an ideal of a matchstick girl without breasts or bum – of which Twiggy was the prime example, one of a score of skinny women who became the role-models for their generation. The outcome has been a vicious circle in which designers, manufacturers, and women's magazines are locked. Thin clothes need thin models – which end up in thin advertisements and on thin fashion pages.

Would-be thin readers, all desperately try to look like the girl in the pictures. These women are the true fashion victims, who don't just squander their hard-earned money on unrealistic diet aids and ephemeral fashion items, but put their health at risk into the bargain.

In an article, "Would You Dare Not to Diet?", published in *Options*, Kathryn Hughes quotes the results of an American magazine survey: ". . . the majority of women place a weight loss of 10–15 lbs (5–7 kilos), at the top of a list of 'Things That Would Make Me Happy' – well above success in love or work". She records a horrifying extension of the dieting urge: the Eating Disorders Unit in London's Great Ormond Street Hospital for Children now treats girls as young as eight, already launched on the starve/binge road to health ruin.

From time to time, fashion editors run a token feature on "Fashion for the Larger Woman" – usually photographed on a size 14 or 16 model 1.78m (5ft 10ins) tall. But few fashion editors can tear themselves away from the false image of Ideal Women they have created. Few manufacturers bother to cater for this "minority" market. Stores rarely give their bigger women customers more than a rail or two of clothes to choose from, usually tucked away into a discreet corner. All this in spite of the fact that one in three women in Britain is overweight, and nearly half the population is a size 14 or over.

Things are changing. In the United States a groundswell of protest is building against the discrimination that sees fat people as failures. "It's time you did something about your weight: accept it" is the battle-cry of the new Liberation movement for fat people. "What we have to change is the cultural myths about fat people – not fat people themselves," says Sally Smith, director of NAAFA, the National Association for the Advancement of Fat Acceptance. NAAFA has branches all over the United States, sends out a spirited monthly newsletter, holds an annual Conference, and challenges employers who discriminate against the obese. A study conducted by the University of Vermont showed that 30 per cent of the fat women surveyed had had promotion denied them because of their excess weight, while 17 per cent had lost their jobs.

Exuberant outsize TV stars Roseanne Barr and Oprah Winfrey have probably helped millions of obese viewers to come to terms with their own dimensions. A crop of new magazines has sprung up to target this huge and neglected market: the most famous is *Bbw*, which stands for Big Beautiful Women. In response to their lobbying, a chain of shops called – aptly – *The Forgotten Woman* – now sells clothes specially designed for outsize customers by famous names like Oscar della Renta: already there are branches in over two dozen American cities.

Even mainstream magazines in Europe and the United States are beginning to reflect a rising resistance to this brainwashing. The British magazine *Woman* now has a firm editorial policy of not using pictures that show ultra-thin models. They even ran a competition to find the best size 16 plus model in Britain, and received over 5,000 entries.

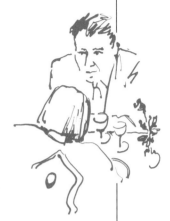

**Fame is no protection against Fattism**

In her article "Food on the Brain", published in *New York Woman*, and *She* in Britain, Elizabeth Gleick took a searching look at what the Diet Obsession actually does to women. She came to the melancholy conclusion: "It's a rare woman who's satisfied with her weight or the way her body looks. Most women, whether they're actively doing anything about it or not, would like to lose 5 to 10 pounds (2–5 kg)". The whole dieting obsession, she concluded, was "a huge burden and a tremendous waste of energy. It's a little terrifying to imagine how many brilliant ideas and how much enjoyment of life are lost, pushed out of mind by thoughts of chips and chocolates, or by pledges to sweat it off". Despite these embryonic changes in attitude, to be fat in Western society today is to be an outcast.

Even fame is no protection against Fattism. What kind of society do we live in when a towering talent like Luciano Pavarotti, owner of perhaps the most beautiful tenor voice in the world, can be brutally snubbed by a salesman. Reportedly he went to an outsize shop and asked what they had to fit him. "A pair of cufflinks?" was the offhand answer. When I (Barbara), went on the Wogan show, superstar Pavarotti was a fellow-guest – and caused huge confusion because he refused to walk on to the set. Pavarotti insisted on being "discovered" already seated behind a protective table that concealed his bulk, such was his fear of ridicule for his excess kilos in a society obsessed with thinness. Fat is not only a feminist issue, as is demonstrated by the growing numbers of young boys now suffering from anorexia.

**Mental torment and nagging hunger pangs are NOT essential to your diet!**

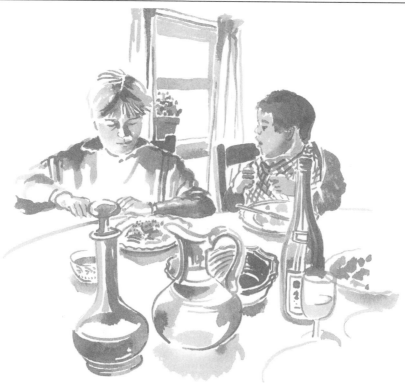

Even worse than the actual miseries of dieting – the pangs of unappeased hunger – is the overwhelming mental torment. Millions of perpetual dieters – mostly women – spend their waking hours literally obsessed by food. One of us (Michael) was consulted by a slim, intelligent woman in her late twenties, 1.67m (5ft 6ins) tall and weighing 54kg (8 st 7lbs). Having spent two years struggling to lose weight and improve her diet, she was still convinced that her "addiction" to sweet biscuits was the reason that she couldn't shed the last few pounds which she felt compelled to do. Expecting to hear that she was eating at least a packet a day, I was stunned when she "confessed" to munching her way through . . . two whole biscuits daily! She wanted help to overcome this "weakness". No amount of persuasion would convince her that far from losing more weight, she should try to gain a few pounds, or that there was any crime in eating a couple of biscuits.

Dieters know by heart the calorie content of almost every food in their local supermarket. They can recite their last week's daily menus, and for them, eating equals guilt. They are strangers to one of the most important ingredients of a balanced diet – pleasure.

CHAPTER 2

# ARE YOU IN GOOD SHAPE?

The perceived medical wisdom is that being fat is unhealthy. This idea has seeped into our collective consciousness, and everyone from prospective employers to insurance companies, from building societies to your family doctor – and even your nearest and dearest – believes this to be the absolute truth. It is, in fact, far from the truth. There is no denying that severe obesity puts your health at risk. You are more likely to suffer from arthritis of the feet, knees, hips, and spine. There is an increased chance of developing diabetes or gallstones in later life. Respiratory disease becomes more common. And if you ever need to have an operation, you become a surgeon's nightmare as the risks rise dramatically with so much surplus fat.

That most popular theory, of the links between excess weight and heart disease, may be the most misleading of them all. Recent research suggests that the consumption of foods that cause overweight rather than the weight itself could be the major factor: if you're fat because your diet is excessively rich in fatty foods, you are likely to have heart disease. If you're fat as a result of eating too many starchy foods, you are not. A severely underweight exercise fanatic who binges on butter, cream, burgers, and chips is at greater risk than the Couch Potato who eats a healthy diet, albeit overgenerous.

Key factors are high blood pressure and raised cholesterol levels. If you are moderately overweight, live on Superfoods, don't smoke, have a modest alcohol intake, and enjoy good health – DON'T WORRY ABOUT YOUR WAISTLINE. Unless you want to look slimmer.

In *Being Fat is Not a Sin*, Shelley Bovey examines attitudes to fatness, and the psychological repercussions of being a fatty in a society that worships thinnies. She has also sifted through a mass of research – much of it completely ignored by the press – that paints a very different picture. Among others, she quotes Dr. Celia Oakley, one of Britain's foremost cardiologists. Asked about the link between heart disease and excess weight, she replied that "if you are overweight but do not have high blood pressure, high blood fats, or diabetes, there is no associated risk".

Dr. Reuben Andres, of the American National Institute of Ageing, reviewed 16 medical studies from the United States and Europe. He concluded, Bovey tells us, that "the major studies of obesity and mortality fail to show that overall obesity leads to greater risk".

A startling study quoted by Bovey, the world's largest ever population survey, monitored 1.8 million Norwegians over a period of 10 years. The highest death rate of all occurred in underweight women: those of 45.3kg (7st 2lbs) and under at 1.6m (5ft 3ins) were twice as likely to die prematurely than those of around 60kg (11st), while even the obese lived longer.

Life expectancy calculations based on the Norwegian study produced some surprising results. The life expectancy of the "fat" women – 1.7m (5ft 6ins) tall, weighing 102.5kg (16st) and over – was actually slightly greater than that of the ideal insurance company candidates – 1.7m (5ft 6ins) and 55.5kg (8st 10lbs); 844 of the "fatties" will survive to age 65, compared to only 824 of the "ideal" women. And even the real heavyweights – 127kg (20st) – should live longer (757 out of a thousand reaching 65) than the group at the highest risk, the "thinnies" who are 1.7m (5ft 6ins) and 50kg (7st 12lbs). A mere 730 – less than 75 per cent – will celebrate their 65th birthday.

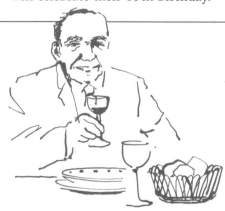

**Your ideal weight for health increases with age**

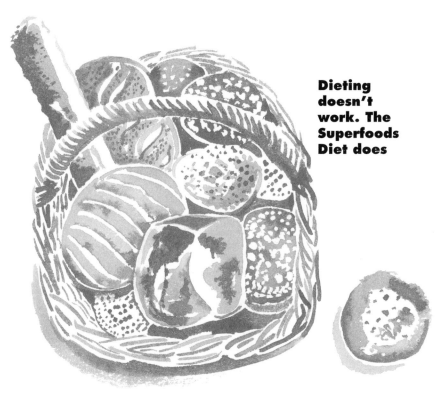

**Dieting doesn't work. The Superfoods Diet does**

In summing up the completely different picture painted by such recent studies in their book, *The Amazing Brain*, Robert Ornstein and Richard F. Thompson conclude that: "In all age and height groups, people who are slightly fat are the healthiest, and the ideal weight for health, increases with age. This increase is almost exactly the amount gained on average".

The Superfoods Diet will enable you to shed any surplus pounds gradually but effortlessly, without ever counting a calorie, without going to bed hungry, or feeling deprived. If you are absolutely certain that you *need* to lose weight urgently, and that this need is consistent with good health and sound sense, then you may find that the quick start weight loss plan on p.47 will get the first pounds off faster, and give you the incentive to make the Superfoods Diet the basis of your everyday eating for life.

CHAPTER 3

# WHY DIETS DON'T WORK

Diets don't work because the very thought of trying yet another wonder regime saps your self-esteem in advance. Before you've got to the end of the first page of that revolutionary diet book, feelings of guilt, self-contempt, and failure are already welling up. You know it won't work. You know that you aren't going to be able to stick with it. You blame yourself for your lack of determination and will-power. The truth is, diets don't work because they're boring, depressing, antisocial, unpleasant, unrealistic, extreme, unworkable, unhealthy, and inflexible. How many of us ever want to go on a diet? We may feel that we need to, we may feel that we ought to, we may feel that others think we ought to, even our doctors may think that we ought to . . . but want to? You must be kidding. All diet books could be subtitled – *I'll Start on Monday*.

In view of the worldwide obsession with weight, it's not surprising that a succession of ill-informed, outrageous, and often frankly dangerous diet books dominate the bestseller lists. A new crop appears every month; their temporary success is as assured as the fact that most of those who buy them will end up fatter than they started.

There were the original low-calorie, low-carbohydrate, high-protein diets – all the doctors wrote those. There was the Drinking Man's Diet, the Champagne Diet, the Grapefruit and Hard-boiled Egg Diet (a gift to all the laxative manufacturers); the All-Fruit Diet (a boon to all the dentists); the High-Fibre Diet (which turned cheap horsefeed into a money-spinner); and the Businessman's Diet (how to get slim on expense accounts).

**Diets that are boring, inflexible, and simply unrealistic don't work**

More recently, there have been the VLC or very-low calorie diets which have actually killed people, and the virtually fat-free diet which claimed to trim specific bits of your anatomy.

Growing ranks of prescription drugs "aid" the unhappy slimmer, as international pharmaceutical companies scramble to board this golden gravy-train. In theory drugs should be prescribed with great restraint for desperate cases; in practice unscrupulous "diet specialists" shell them out freely to their wealthy overweight clients.

Amphetamine-derived appetite suppressors can give you high blood pressure, insomnia, and nervous problems: you can get hooked on these. So-called thermogenic drugs theoretically up your metabolic rate to increase calorie expenditure. Based on thyroid, growth, or sex hormones, they can be highly toxic, with high blood pressure, high or low blood sugar, cardiac problems, thyroid disfunction, insulin problems, irritability, depression, and migraine among possible scary side effects. Enzyme-inhibiting drugs work "naturally" by reducing the absorption of fats and sugars: they're dangerous because a number of

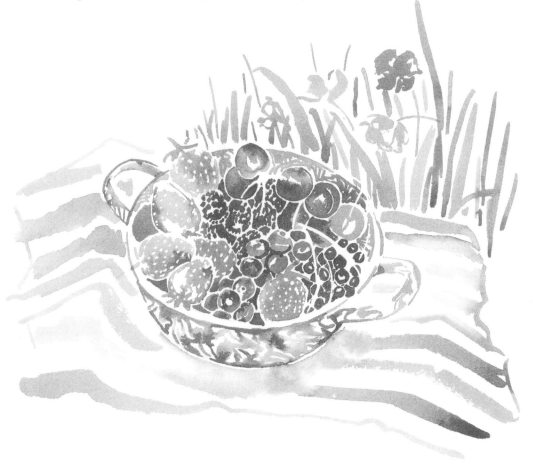

vital nutrients are contained in fats, and some fats themselves are essential. There are the laxatives and diuretics, many of them herbal, that cause a temporary drop in weight – but flush out vital nutrients, too.

We've had the Raw Food Diet, the Macrobiotic Diet, the Gourmet Diet, and the Rotation Diet. And now, finally, the wheel has come full circle. One of the newest books on the market extols the virtues of low-calorie, high-protein eating.

In his book *The Sensible Person's Guide to Weight Control*, John Yudkin, Emeritus Professor of Nutrition at London University, discusses what he describes as "nonsense diet books". He claims that "many of them give dietary advice that, if followed for any length of time, would lead to malnutrition, sometimes quite severe; luckily, the diets they describe are so ridiculous, so difficult to follow, and often so costly, that it is not long before they are abandoned, at least until the next crazy diet book appears".

How many of them have you tried? How many times in your life have you followed the latest fad? You stuck it heroically for a week – lost five pounds – and then gave up the struggle to stick with an impossibly draconian diet. You promptly gained seven pounds. This is the nightmare of the yo-yo dieter, a pattern familiar to millions of people, especially women.

The yo-yo dieter is trapped in a lifelong obsession with food: on a diet, struggling to stay with a diet, giving up a diet – and starting a new diet after a guilt-ridden binge. Always seeking the easy, miracle answer to weight problems, and always finding that each new regime brings its own problems. So low in calories that energy vanishes faster than the pounds; so high in fibre that the antisocial flatulence becomes unbearable; so lacking in nerve nutrients that tempers fray; and so totally devoid of enjoyment that mealtimes become a misery.

Another reason why diets don't work is the difference between what people think they're eating, and what they actually eat. American archeologists have recently become interested in "garbology" – the study of modern garbage. Using core extractors, they have looked at infill sites around the United States and come up with startling insights into the American Way of Eating. Dating their samples by newspapers, they tell us that when the United States Health Authorities began recommending reducing fat intake to avoid bowel cancer, garbage tips filled with trimmed-off surplus fat from steaks, chops, roasts, and slices of bacon. Within weeks, wrappers from sausages, salamis, bologna, and luncheon meats appeared: consumption of hidden fats had zoomed.

The next exhortation from the Government was to eat more green vegetables for their protective effect against cancer. Sales in the shops rocketed as every mother determined to feed these wonderfoods to her family. Sadly, a huge percentage of these sales ended up in the rubbish tip uneaten. Good intentions didn't get as far as the dinner-table.

Most of us like to think that we eat lots of good things, cut down on the unhealthy things, and drink only sensible amounts of alcohol. Garbologists know better. When questioned, most people over-report their consumption of fresh fruit, vegetables, and salads, and play down their alcohol intake. Here is your chance to face up to reality: keep a diet diary for a week. If it goes in your mouth, write it down. Keep the diary honestly – after all, you'll only be cheating yourself; don't change the way you eat and drink – that's cheating too. We have looked at thousands of diet diaries; and we can promise you that nearly everyone who does is in for a shock.

Yo-yo dieting isn't just a crazy way to live. It can seriously damage your health – and does. A number of studies have shown that inevitably, over the years, weight creeps up on this stop-start regime. Research is slowly revealing the intricate feedback mechanisms by which the hypothalamus, the master-gland of the brain, regulates your intake of food and keeps it in nutritional balance. But the brain cannot function efficiently without a steady supply of sugar. This does not mean that we all need spoonfuls of sugar in our tea, or bars of chocolate in our pockets.

The body's chemistry creates sugar in the form that it needs from fats, proteins, and carbohydrates. If you eat a balanced diet, this sugar is gradually released into the bloodstream – natural, or added sugar from food getting there first, followed by sugar from the digestion of complex carbohydrates (whole grains and vegetables), followed by sugars from fats and finally proteins. What makes it worse is that the surplus fat moves gradually up the body. If you eat a large amount of sugar and refined carbohydrates at the same time, there will be an almost instant surge in the amount of sugar circulating in the

**Face up to reality by keeping an honest Diet Diary and prepare yourself for a shock**

bloodstream. The pancreas will pump out insulin to destroy it, and the sugar levels will tumble. Unfortunately, the pancreas doesn't always know when to stop. It is often a step or two behind the real sugar-levels. Consequently too much sugar is destroyed, and the blood-sugar level falls so far that the brain sends urgent messages demanding more sugar. You reach for the bar of chocolate, sweet tea or coffee, digestive biscuits, and the sugar bowl. You are instantly trapped in a vicious circle of worse and worse nutrition, and more and more surplus pounds.

Professor Judith Stern, an American professor of Nutrition, told us of her research, which should encourage every woman not to fight against her genetic inheritance. The common European pear-shape, in which any surplus fat tends to concentrate around the hips, is certainly preferable to being barrel-shaped, when fat deposits form around the waist and upper body. Pear-shaped overweight types are less at risk of heart disease than their barrel-shaped counterparts of the same weight. Any pear who consistently loses and then regains weight will gradually turn into a barrel. Far from achieving their desired objective of becoming slimmer, they suffer all the miseries of constant dieting, stay the same weight or more, change their body shape, and increase their risk of contracting heart disease.

Use a tape-measure to calculate your stomach–hips ratio. Measure yourself first around the belly-button, and then around the widest part of your hips. Divide the belly-button measurement by the hip-measurement (borrow your child's calculator if you can't do long division). For women the answer should be 0.75 or less; for men, 1.0 or less. If your ratio exceeds these figures, your risk of heart disease goes up.

Boredom and misery are not the whole story of why diets don't work. They don't work because they can't work. Your own body takes very good care that they don't. You are biologically programmed for survival; and the wisdom of the body perceives dieting as starvation; a threat to be actively – and successfully – countered.

Recent research into the brain and nervous system has made it clear that eating, like breathing, is an activity directly controlled by the brain. Situated within the hypothalamus are clusters of cells that exercise a regulatory function over our weight, partly by controlling appetite, and partly by adjusting our metabolic rate – the speed at which calories burn to produce energy. Regulating cells collectively known as the *appestat* work against almost every weight-loss diet. Their objective, to ensure that you eat when your body needs nourishment, and stop only when those needs are met, is not yours.

When you start that amazing new low-calorie Three-Day Wonder Diet you read about in your favourite magazine, the appestat goes into action. A sharp drop in your food intake leads to a slow-down in your metabolic rate, designed to conserve energy, and responsible for the fatigue that goes with low-calorie dieting. This also explains the other phenomenon familiar to every dieter – the law of diminishing returns. The less food you eat, the less weight you lose. When you stop dieting and return to normal eating (or go on a reckless binge), your metabolism will still be running at the low, emergency, rate. You will put on more weight than before.

When the appestat mechanism is disordered or damaged, body weight can fluctuate wildly. Experimental animals which had had certain clusters of midbrain cells destroyed – rats, mice, dogs, and cats among them – began bingeing and became obese. When other groups of cells were damaged, they stopped eating and starved to death.

Diets that work against the natural function of the appestat mechanism are doomed to fail. "The secret of avoiding obesity does not . . . lie in the avoidance of either fat or carbohydrate, but in providing oneself with the full nutritional chain of life," points out Roger Williams. ". . . Fighting obesity without Nature's help – without adequate appestat mechanism – is like travelling up a swift-flowing river in a row-boat. Nature's way of preventing obesity needs to be understood and utilized". If dieting is so futile – and so dangerous – then why have we written another diet book? We'll answer that question in the next chapter.

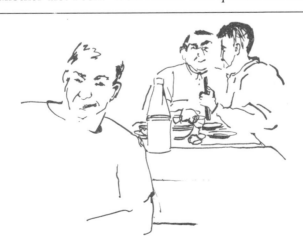

**Diets that oppose the natural function of the body's appestat mechanism are doomed to fail**

C H A P T E R  4

# THE SUPERFOODS DIET

We promised we would answer your question: if we're so sure that diets don't work – why are we writing a diet book? The answer is because this is not a "diet" in the accepted modern sense of the word – a rigid and wretched regime of undereating for the sole purpose of losing weight, with no consideration for health. What we mean when we talk about diet is the dictionary definition of the word: *a way of eating*.

- A way of eating that is healthy, pleasant, enjoyable, and satisfying.

- A way of eating that can even be just a little self-indulgent: hot, buttered toast and sticky buns for tea. Cream on your strawberries. A glass of claret with your steak. A piece of wonderfully runny Brie.

- A way of eating that says, "It's how you eat most of the time that matters, not how you eat occasionally".

- A way of eating on which you will feel fit, well, and full of energy.

- A way of eating that has a delightful side-effect: if you need to, you will lose weight.

- A way of eating that works for millions of ordinary, sensible people – although it's not for the health fanatics, the cranks or the food obsessives and certainly not for the hair-shirt brigade.

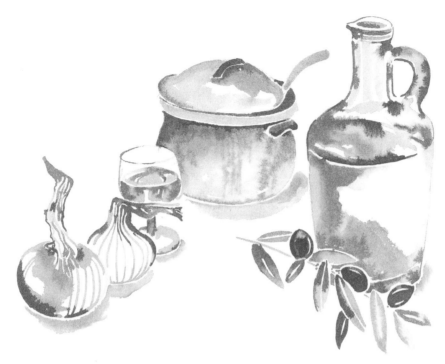

**Hay's diet improved the health of millions throughout the world**

The man who made this way of eating famous – over half a century ago – was an American doctor called William Howard Hay. He developed the system as a solution to his own problem. And his problem, initially, was – excess weight.

As a young man, Dr. Hay tipped the scales at a generous 16 stone or approximately 102kg. One summer he decided to tackle the problem together with a dentist friend. For four months, they closed their surgeries at teatime, and spent a couple of hours playing a vigorous game of tennis. By mutual agreement, neither man weighed himself until the four months was up. They both felt terrific, reported Hay, "with greatly increased endurance and fine appetites".

When Dr. Hay finally weighed himself, he had a disagreeable surprise. He had lost precisely one pound. Disgusted, he chucked the daily game of tennis. The "fine" appetite, however, remained. Within a year his weight had rocketed, and he was suffering from high blood pressure, serious kidney disease, and an enlarged heart.

In desperation, he embarked on a dietary revolution, which was almost certainly inspired by his study of the early American naturopaths and their work. After three months of eating "fundamentally" – the basis of the Superfoods Diet, too – his health was completely recovered, he had lost nearly 25kg (4st), he was able to run long distances, and he felt years younger.

When he put his patients on the same diet, Hay reported "many cases of supposedly incurable disease that have recovered completely". All of his patients told him that "their health is now at the highest point it has ever attained".

Hay's rules for happy eating – explained in his bestseller *A New Health Era* – were simplicity itself. Don't mix foods that fight – never eat concentrated starches and proteins at the same meal. Eat fats, starches, sugar, and proteins only in small amounts; make vegetables and fruit 80 per cent of your diet; avoid refined starches and sugars altogether.

The book was published in Britain in 1935, and among its earliest fans was Doris Grant, a young woman in her twenties. She claims to have cured herself of severe rheumatism in just four weeks. Astonished and impressed, she wrote a series of articles on the diet for a Sunday newspaper. Hundreds of letters poured in to the newspaper's offices, and direct to Doris Grant, when she followed up the articles with a cookery book called *The Hay Diet*.

Readers told how the Hay system of compatible eating had changed their lives almost overnight, clearing their minds, banishing weight problems, ending the urge for between-meals snacks, and improving overall health to a quite astonishing extent.

In 1939, Hay's diet came by chance to the attention of a young German physician, Dr. Ludwig Walb, who was already experimenting with a number of the dietary therapies then being advocated. He tried it out on a nine-year-old boy suffering from advanced kidney disease for which conventional medicine could offer no cure. To his amazement, Hay's regime brought an almost immediate improvement, and eventually a cure. At the clinic he set up in Ohm after the war, Dr. Walb and his wife and partner, Dr. Ilse Walb, adopted the Hay regime as standard treatment, and found that cardiac problems, diabetes, gout, rheumatism, asthma, and digestive disorders were among the long list of diseases that were strikingly alleviated and often completely cured by the adoption of this diet alone.

Summing up the results of a number of clinical studies, Walb concluded that the Hay regime worked to improve the digestion, normalize the metabolism, and promote the efficient function of both mind and body. Almost in passing, he noted that on the Hay diet, body weight became normal.

The Walb-Hay book has been a steady bestseller in Germany since the late 1950s, producing a stream of grateful letters from readers. Even in Italy – where dozens of popular pasta dishes with their combinations of starch, meat, and cheese are Hay non-starters – a translation of Walb's work, with plenty of Italian-style recipes, has run through 20 printings in just four years. And in France, *la cuisine dissociée* may be said to have outlived *la nouvelle cuisine*.

Throughout Europe, indeed, the number of converts to this simple way of healthy eating, with its immediate bonus of improved well-being, has turned into a flood. The younger members of the Royal Family attribute their slimline looks and glowing good health to the Hay regime.

The Hay system has been the subject of a number of scientific studies, chiefly in Germany, but just exactly how and why it works is still something of a medical mystery.

There are, however, many precedents for using successful treatments for which there is as yet no rational explanation – if they work, and if they cause no harm, why not?

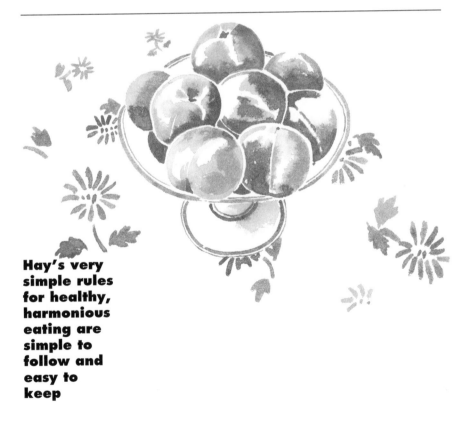

**Hay's very simple rules for healthy, harmonious eating are simple to follow and easy to keep**

**It's never too late to change your eating habits for the better**

We offer this Superfoods regime without excuse or explanation, except to say that we know it works. We are confident, however, that scientific research will sooner or later establish a rationale for the Hay regime. Already there are significant clues. One clue was supplied by Dr. Roger Williams, one of the world's most outstanding biochemists and a pioneer researcher into the links between nutrition and disease. He writes that "as a result of studies designed to clear the milk-tolerance problem, it has been found that healthy adult individuals have in their intestinal mucosa widely varying amounts of lactase, which digests lactose, but also widely varying amounts of sucrase, which digests ordinary sugar, and maltase, which splits malt sugar. These variations, among a group of 100 healthy individuals, were in each case 10- to 20-fold or more".

"If these carbohydrate-digesting enzymes vary so enormously from one well individual to another, how can we escape the probability that other digestive enzymes vary in the same manner in *normal* people?" (Dr. Roger Williams, *Nutrition Against Disease*)

This being so, it is not unreasonable to expect enormous variations in individual ability to deal with different foods and food combinations. The beauty of the Superfoods Diet is that – unlike nearly all other regimes – it does not depend on the exclusion of important and highly nutritious food groups. It simply separates them from each other, and allows a full spectrum of nutrients to be consumed in a manner that seems to allow for greater efficiency of digestion.

Significantly, the Hay regime is particularly successful for a number of problems known to result from food allergies, such as eczema, rheumatoid disorders, asthma, hay fever, migraine, and fatigue.

People embarking on this way of eating for the first time almost invariably report the disappearance of digestive disturbances, and a new ease and comfort throughout the whole digestive system. Since improved digestion means an improved intake of nutrients from what we eat, we may logically surmise that our appestats – like every other bodily function – will also work more efficiently when they are supplied with the full spectrum of nourishment.

"The cells in the mid-brain that constitute the appestat mechanism are like other cells in our bodies", observed Roger Williams. "They have definite functions, and if they are provided with a good environment, the chances are excellent that they will do a good job. . . . We need to concentrate on the health of the appestat mechanisms instead of calorie counting and the sheer exercise of will-power."

Suggestive proof that the Superfoods Diet can make your appestat more efficient is provided by the fact that people following it almost invariably report that the urge to binge – that downfall of every ordinary diet – has disappeared.

The Superfoods Diet will provide you – and your appestat – with a cornucopia of top-quality nutrition in delicious recipes. Far from being deprived of nutrients when you follow this way of eating, your diet will contain a greater abundance of all the essential vitamins, proteins, trace elements, fats, proteins, and carbohydrates than you have ever enjoyed before.

Don't begin to put this book down while you decide to "start on Monday": turn the page, read the rules, and start right now. You have nothing to lose but your surplus pounds – and nothing to gain but good health.

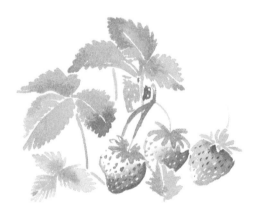

C H A P T E R   5

# THE SEVEN GOLDEN RULES

There are seven simple, basic rules for the Superfoods Diet. Here they are:

### RULE ONE: EAT SUPERFOODS

Superfoods are all the good, natural, wholesome foodstuffs that have successfully nourished the human race for millennia. Superfoods are the succulent fruits, the freshest of vegetables, the crispest of salads. They are sea-fresh fish, naturally reared poultry, game, beef, and lamb; wholegrains, nuts, seeds, pulses, and cold-pressed oils; good cheeses, butter, milk, cream, and yogurt; savoury herbs and aromatic spices.

The Superfoods have the best flavours, the best textures, and the highest nutritional values. Many of them also have specific protective and healing properties – as we described in our book *Superfoods*.

### RULE TWO: EAT REGULARLY

Successful weight loss depends on regular eating, not stuffing one day and starving the next, and certainly not starving all day and stuffing late in the evening. Aim to eat properly balanced meals – although not necessarily large ones – at regular intervals.

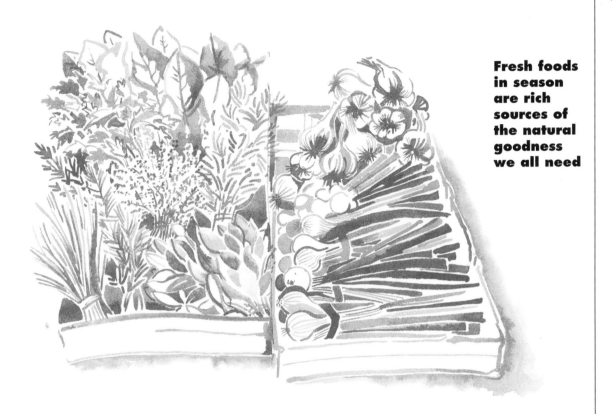

**Fresh foods in season are rich sources of the natural goodness we all need**

### RULE THREE: EAT FRESH FOODS IN SEASON

Wherever possible, eat fruit and vegetables in their appropriate season, and better still, those grown on your own doorstep. They will be more likely to have been harvested at their peak of perfection; and they will have lost fewer nutrients sitting around in storage or transportation.

Exotic fruits and strange tropical vegetables — for all their high nutritional value and wonderful flavours — are often chemically treated to ripen them artificially in transit.

### RULE FOUR: AVOID POOR FOODS

Poor Foods are the high-fat, high-sugar, refined and processed products of the giant food-manufacturing industries: the pastries and the biscuits, the sweets and the chocolates, the sugary breakfast cereals, the pies, the pâtés and the luncheon meats, the high-fat salty snacks-in-a-packet, the just-add-milk desserts, and the ice-cream gâteaux. These are not just the enemies of your figure, but of your health too. Don't use white flour; use wholemeal. Eat brown rice instead of white — or if you find it tedious to cook with, at least pick parboiled rice, which has many of its nutrients steam-processed into the white starchy centre before hulling to avoid some nutrient losses.

### RULE FIVE: EAT HARMONIOUSLY

The chart opposite shows you what to eat with what. All foods belong in one of three food groups. Protein. Neutral. Or Starch. You can eat Neutral Foods with any of the Protein Foods or with any of the Starch Foods, BUT NEVER EAT PROTEIN FOODS AND STARCH FOODS AT THE SAME MEAL.

Aim to eat one Starch meal, one Protein meal, and one meal composed mainly of fruits, vegetables and salads each day, with yogurt if you like it.

Allow four hours between Starch and Protein Meals. If you are overcome by the urge to snack in between, try to stick to Neutral foods. If you had a Starch lunch at 1pm, and hunger gnaws you at 4pm – you could have Neutral or Starch foods: perhaps a banana, or one of our little Raisin Buns (p.157) with your cup of tea. But if you are planning a Protein evening meal at 8pm, and you want a nibble at 6.30pm – stick to Neutral or Protein: a few black olives, or a sliver of cheese. Once you have been on the Diet for a week or two, however, you will probably find that the urge to nibble between meals has magically disappeared.

### RULE SIX: EAT MODERATELY

You don't need a pair of scales and a magnifying glass to follow the Superfoods Diet. You won't be weighing out cheese by the gram, or counting up the number of grapes in a bunch. But a little self-control is called for. If it's a Starch meal, for instance, by all means enjoy a slice or two of wholemeal bread with that thick vegetable soup – and a little butter with it. But don't go on to finish off the loaf – or empty the butter-dish. Enjoy a glass of wine with your Protein dinner on a special occasion – but not three or four. If your self-control fails on any occasion – and of course it will – don't worry. Don't give up. Just pick up the Superfoods Diet again at the next meal.

### RULE SEVEN: EAT CALMLY AND SLOWLY

Breakfast bolted with an eye on the clock, rushed sandwich lunches at your desk, Fast Food gulped down as you go, meals eaten when you're feeling tired and frazzled: they're all death to good digestion. And a happy digestive system is what the Superfoods Diet is about. Take time to sit down to your meal, eat slowly, and enjoy it.

## WHAT TO EAT WITH WHAT

| PROTEIN | NEUTRAL | STARCH |
|---|---|---|
| Meat<br>Poultry<br>Game<br>Fish<br>Shellfish<br>Eggs (whole)<br>Cheese | All vegetables except potatoes,<br>yams, and sweetcorn | Potatoes<br>Yams<br>Sweetcorn |
| All fruits except those in the<br>starch group | All nuts except peanuts | Bread<br>Flour<br>Oats<br>Wheat<br>Barley<br>Rice<br>Millet<br>Rye<br>Buckwheat |
| All dried fruits except raisins,<br>which are neutral | Butter<br>Cream<br>Cream cheese (see note**)<br>Ricotta cheese<br>Egg yolks | |
| Tomatoes (see note*) | Yogurt and milk:<br>these are protein foods, but<br>their protein content is low,<br>and they can be used IN VERY<br>SMALL AMOUNTS ONLY<br>with starch foods | Very sweet fruits such as<br>Ripe pears<br>Bananas<br>Papaya<br>Mango<br>Very sweet grapes |
| Peanuts | | |
| Soya beans<br>Tofu | Cold-pressed sesame, sunflower,<br>or olive oils | Beer |
| Milk<br>Yogurt<br>All cheeses except cream cheese<br>and ricotta cheese | All salad stuffs | |
| | Lentils, dried split peas, dried or<br>canned beans, chickpeas, etc,<br>but not soya beans<br>(see note***) | |
| Wine<br>Cider | Seeds and sprouted seeds | |
| | Herbs and spices<br>Raisins | |
| | Honey and maple syrup | |

### NOTES

*When tomatoes are cooked, they undergo chemical changes that increase their acidity, and make them unsuitable for consumption with starch foods.

**Cream cheese contains only small amounts of protein, so it is classed as neutral. Because of its very high (nearly 50 per cent) fat content – it should be used sparingly on the Superfoods Diet. So easily digested that it may be considered neutral, ricotta is technically a protein food.

***Legumes such as lentils, dried beans, and dried peas contain substantial amounts of both starch and protein, so they are harder to digest than other foods, and should be eaten only occasionally on the Superfoods Diet, where they are treated, for this reason, as a neutral food. For vegetarians, however, they are an important source of protein.

CHAPTER 6

# THE SUPERFOODS DIET IN PRACTICE

Working out what to eat with what may take a week or two but you'll soon become practised at planning ahead, and juggling Starch and Protein meals to take into account invitations out, birthdays, business lunches, picnics, and other special occasions. To help you get it all together, we've drawn up menus for a week's Harmonious Eating in spring, summer, autumn, and winter, using the recipes in the second part of the book. We have also suggested menus for Special Occasions, for Vegetarian meals, and for easy Packed Lunches. You don't have to stick to these menus, obviously, although you may find it helpful to do so at first.

Studying these menus, you may find it hard to believe you could actually lose weight on them. But you will be surprised to find that excess weight starts disappearing slowly but steadily, even when you are eating foods that would be off-limits on any "normal" diet: hot, crusty rolls with butter and honey, for instance. The fact remains — as thousands of people have been surprised and delighted to discover — that you will lose weight. You may feel dismally that almost every Protein meal has a big starch-shaped hole in it, and wonder how you will ever get used to meat without potatoes, or no roll when you're eating soup. Don't worry: just try it.

You will notice that most meals in our menus begin with a salad or simple raw vegetable dish. There's good evidence that starting a meal with raw fruit or vegetables pre-programmes your digestion to extra efficiency — and it certainly cuts your appetite. This good habit will also increase your efficient intake of the wonder-working Superfoods.

When you look at our menus, you will be struck by the amount of fruit and fresh vegetables they feature. You may well wonder if your housekeeping budget isn't going to be severely stretched. You will also notice that although these menus are certainly not for vegetarians, they feature very little red meat – always the heaviest item in any weekly budget. Instead, there are recipes for fish, chicken, turkey, and rabbit – all of which are not just healthier foods, lower in saturated fats, but cheaper into the bargain. Eating locally grown Superfoods in season is much cheaper than eating whatever you fancy all the year round: in January, for instance, carrots and cabbage are daily bargains, while you could be paying a small fortune for imported baby courgettes or early peas.

You will certainly be surprised to see cream featured in a number of recipes and menus – excepting those for Intensive Weight Loss. In fact, the amounts used are relatively small – we certainly don't recommend heaping double whipped cream on to puddings. We use it mainly to add texture, interest, and pleasure to eating. The extra calories are more than offset by the small amounts of high-fat meat or complex made-up dishes you'll be eating.

You may worry, too, about the amount of time you are likely to spend cleaning and trimming vegetables, and preparing salads – a great feature of the Superfoods Diet. But you will be saving time too: few of our recipes are particularly complicated, or require great

**Locally grown Superfoods in season are cheap, tasty, and nutritious**

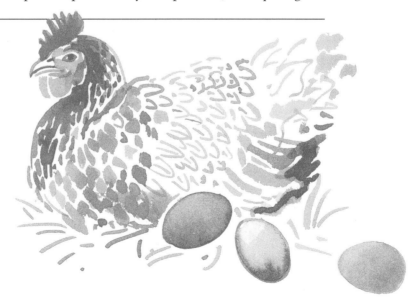

**Start your meals with fruit or raw vegetables**

numbers of ingredients. In general, you will find yourself eating much more simply. When shopping, for instance, you'll find yourself studying what Superfoods are available fresh and in season, and planning your meals around them, rather than studying endless cookery books, and planning dishes that call for exotic ingredients. In the recipe section, we have included a number of recipes for vegetarian dishes. But most of the time, vegetables should be cooked as simply and as briefly as possible.

The Superfoods Diet obviously works best when you stick to it. But you don't have to be 100 per cent rigid 100 per cent of the time. There's room for just a little licence in the way you interpret the rules. Milk, for instance, is a Protein food – but a little in your cup of tea with a starchy breakfast is fine. Lemon juice is an acid food that doesn't harmonize with Starch – but a salad isn't a salad to us without at least a touch of lemon or vinegar in the dressing. Yogurt is a Protein food: but a spoonful stirred into a Starch dish that three or four people will share won't wreck your diet either.

Everybody enjoys the occasional sticky bun, bar of chocolate, or take-away snack. There are moments when we all feel the need for a treat, and the diet that doesn't allow for an occasional luxury is unrealistic: a moment of indulgence certainly does NOT mean you should give up on the Superfoods Diet. Just enjoy your treat – *harmoniously*: chocolates, sweets, sticky buns, and french fries should not be eaten within four hours of a Protein meal, for instance; or a chunk of cheese just an hour after a sandwich lunch. You can pick up Harmonious Eating at the next meal.

We are certainly not suggesting that you can slip into the baker's shop or the corner sweet shop whenever you feel like it. On the Superfoods Diet, you probably won't even want to, after a while. The more Superfoods you eat, the less you'll suffer from those dramatic peaks and plunges in blood-sugar levels which result in sugar cravings, eating binges, and the mood swings that drive you to the biscuit tin or the bottle.

The downfall of most diets can be eating out on special occasions such as birthdays or anniversaries, or just to be sociable, with friends. You're now into the second week of your Superfoods Diet, for instance; you planned a simple Starch Supper – and a friend who's a gourmet cook asks you to an impromptu feast. So what do you do? Accept with pleasure, of course, enjoy every mouthful – and start again. You can't "blow" the Superfoods Diet with one meal out.

You may find it tough at first to say goodbye to familiar food combinations. You may find it odd eating cheese without bread or biscuits, meat without potatoes, fish without chips, roast beef without Yorkshire pudding. You may miss apple tart and spaghetti bolognese, steak and kidney pie and scrambled eggs on toast. But these are items you've probably crossed off the menu dozens of times as you embarked on yet another diet. Now you can enjoy cheese, scrambled eggs, roast beef, and even bread, potatoes, and toast – complete with butter.

On the Superfoods Diet, you can enjoy royal feasts, delicious dinners, tasty snacks, and hearty breakfasts. If you think that's just another example of diet-book hype – turn to p.46 and look at the Special Occasion menus. Most diets are about not eating. On the Superfoods Diet, you'll eat better than ever before.

*Bon Appetit!*

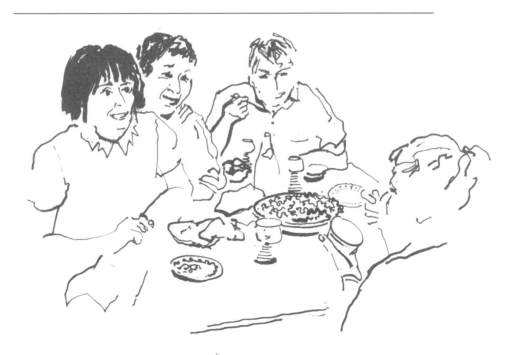

# SPRING

## MONDAY

### Breakfast
Sliced blood oranges, and pink grapefruit segments.
A helping of creamy yogurt, with nuts and honey, if liked.

### Light meal or snack
Tossed Green Salad (p.121).
Scrambled Eggs with Ricotta Cheese (p.87).
Green Beans Parmigiano (p.112).

### Main meal
Sticks of celery and young carrots.
Peppers Stuffed with Rice (p.134).
Spring greens. Green cabbage.
Dates and figs.

## TUESDAY

### Breakfast
Dried Fruit Compôte (p.136), with 1tbs yogurt. An orange.

### Light meal or snack
Lettuce and watercress salad.
Potato and Mushroom Casserole (p.118).
A ripe sweet pear.

### Main meal
Slices of fennel with olive oil, lemon, and a little chopped fresh parsley.
Mustard-marinated Salmon (p.91).
Puréed spinach.
Stewed Apples with Ginger (p.155).

## WEDNESDAY

### Breakfast
Hot wholewheat rolls with butter.
A banana.

### Light meal or snack
Fruit and Cheese Salad (p.125).
An apple.

### Main meal
Aubergine Caviar (p.68) with raw vegetables – carrot, celery, cucumber, fennel, and sprigs of cauliflower.
Turkey Breast with Lemon and White Wine (p.104).
Green beans.

## THURSDAY

### Breakfast
An orange. ½ pink grapefruit.
Yogurt with honey and nuts.

### Light meal or snack
Red Salad (p.130) on lettuce leaves.
Baked potato with 1tbs of ricotta cheese, and plenty of finely chopped fresh herbs.
A ripe sweet pear.

### Main meal
Meze (p.78).
Rosalind's Rabbit with Prunes (p.99).
A purée of young turnips.
Green cabbage cooked *al dente*.
Raisins and nuts.

## FRIDAY

### Breakfast
A sliced sweet pear with 1tbs single cream, raisins, and almonds.

### Light meal or snack
½ avocado pear, sliced, with cress, tomatoes, and cucumber, on a bed of lettuce with a dressing made from 1tbs of olive oil, 2 or 3 drops of lemon juice, seasoning, and chopped fresh herbs.
A crusty wholewheat roll and a little butter.

### Main meal
Beetroot and Apple Soup (p.72).
Fish in a Fiery Sauce (p.90).
Steamed broccoli.
A green salad with watercress.

## SATURDAY

### Breakfast
An orange. An apple. Yogurt.

### Light meal or snack
A big mixed salad, including lettuce, celery, grated carrot, cucumber, tomatoes, watercress, radishes, walnuts, raisins, chopped spring onions, finely chopped garlic, and Sour Cream Dressing I (p.127)
Rye crispbread with cream cheese.
Raisins and nuts.

### Main meal
Cucumber and Watercress Salad (p.131).
Chicken with Onions (p.102).
Steamed spring greens.
Spiced Apricots (p.153). (Make enough for 2 meals.)

## SUNDAY

### Breakfast
Apple juice.
Cold Spiced Apricots (p.153).
Yogurt.

### Light meal or snack
Black Olive Pâté (p.147) with toasted rye bread.
Cucumber and Watercress Salad (p.131).

### Main meal
Aubergine and Tomato Salad (p.69).
Lamb Chop with Tarragon and Cucumber (p.106).
Steamed broccoli.
Orange Soufflé Omelette (p.152).

# SUMMER

## MONDAY

**Breakfast**

Yogurt with slices of nectarine and peach.

**Light meal or snack**

Salad of avocado, cottage cheese, cucumber, black olives, tomatoes, cress, and fresh basil on lettuce. Cold chicken (left over from Sunday) or cottage cheese.

**Main meal**

Lettuce and Pea Soup (p.83). Raw Vegetable Risotto (p.137). Steamed baby courgettes, served with a little olive oil and plenty of chopped parsley.

## TUESDAY

**Breakfast**

A banana. 2 slices of wholewheat toast and butter.

**Light meal or snack**

Salade Niçoise (p.70). A peach.

**Main meal**

½ avocado on shredded lettuce, with a dressing made of olive oil, lemon juice, seasoning, and finely chopped fresh herbs. Salt-fried Sardines (p.92). Green Beans with Garlic and Chilli (p.113).

## WEDNESDAY

**Breakfast**

A lightly boiled egg. A peach.

**Light meal or snack**

A big mixed salad, with plenty of green leaves, including any of the various kinds of lettuce, young spinach, young dandelion leaves, and French Dressing II (p.132). A plate of new potatoes boiled in their skins, with a little butter. Steamed young courgettes.

**Main meal**

Tomato Salad (p.129), served with young spinach or lettuce leaves. Turkey Tonnato (p.103). Lightly steamed baby turnips, and carrots tossed in butter with plenty of chopped parsley. A bunch of grapes.

## THURSDAY

**Breakfast**

A bowl of strawberries, raspberries, and red or black currants. Greek yogurt.

**Light meal or snack**

A green salad – include young spinach or dandelion leaves, and plenty of chopped fresh parsley, watercress or cress. Pasta with Tomato, Garlic and Basil Sauce (p.140).

**Main meal**

Mediterranean Carrot Salad (p.121). Frittata Provençale (p.85). Purée of spinach. Fresh fruit.

## FRIDAY

**Breakfast**

2 or 3 ripe apricots. A small bunch of grapes.

**Light meal or snack**

Pan Bagna (p.150), and a big iceberg lettuce salad, with plenty of cress, cucumber, and Sour Cream Dressing II (p.132).

**Main meal**

Crudités (p.142). Cold Poached Fish (p.94) with Lemon and Yogurt Sauce (p.95). Peas with Lettuce (p.113).

## SATURDAY

**Breakfast**

A ripe sweet pear. A wholewheat roll with butter.

**Light meal or snack**

Avocado, Tomato, and Mushroom Salad (p.126). Courgette Croquettes (p.145).

**Main meal**

A big green salad: rocket, young spinach, dandelion leaves, watercress, any type of lettuce, slivers of cucumber, radishes, plenty of chopped fresh herbs, and an oil and lemon dressing. Baked Tomato Gratin (p.107). Lightly steamed carrots. Peaches in White Wine with Preserved Ginger (p.155).

## SUNDAY

**Breakfast**

A feast of melon – try to have slices of 2 or 3 different kinds.

**Light meal or snack**

Tossed Green Salad (p.121) with French Dressing II (p.132). Onion Quiche (p.147). Fresh beans and broad beans. Sliced sweet pears with raisins, slivers of almond, and a little single cream.

**Main meal**

Nectarine and Pink Grapefruit on Lettuce with Sour Cream Dressing (p.68). Red-hot Chicken (p.100). Purée of Turnips and Carrots (p.115). Green beans. Gooseberry and Elderflower Fool (p.153).

# *AUTUMN*

## MONDAY

**Breakfast**
A peach or a nectarine.
Creamy yogurt.

**Light meal or snack**
Tossed Green Salad (p.121) with
French Dressing II (p.132).
Henri's Mushroom Ragout with
Rice (p.135).
Raisins and nuts.

**Main meal**
Sticks of raw carrot, cucumber,
and celery.
Rustic Frittata (p.84) with spinach.
Stewed Apples with Ginger (p.155).
(Make enough for 2 meals.)

## TUESDAY

**Breakfast**
½ grapefruit. Cold Stewed Apples
with Ginger (p.155).
Yogurt.

**Light meal or snack**
Red Radicchio and Chicory Salad
(p.130) with French Dressing II
(p.132).
Rice, Artichoke, and Potato
Minestrone (p.82) with plenty of
chopped fresh parsley.
Granary bread and butter.
A ripe sweet pear.

**Main meal**
Sticks of raw carrot, celery,
and cucumber.
Lemon-marinated Sardines (p.92).
Green Beans with Garlic and
Chilli (p.113).
Baked Apples with
Blackberries (p.152).

## WEDNESDAY

**Breakfast**
Muesli (p.151) with a very ripe pear.

**Light meal or snack**
A serving of ricotta cheese, with
sliced ripe tomatoes, cucumber, half
an avocado pear, some thinly sliced
mushrooms, plenty of fresh chopped
herbs, and French Dressing II
(p.132).
Raisins and nuts.

**Main meal**
Tomatoes Stuffed with Celery,
Avocado, and Mayonnaise (p.145),
served on a bed of shredded lettuce.
Stuffed Courgettes (p.108).
Green cabbage.

## THURSDAY

**Breakfast**
A big bunch of grapes.
Yogurt with nuts and honey.

**Light meal or snack**
Tossed Green Salad (p.12).
Baked potato with sour cream and
fresh herbs.
A ripe sweet pear.

**Main meal**
Fennel and Watercress Salad (p.131).
Stir-fried Turkey Breast with Celery,
Walnuts, and Oranges (p.104).
Steamed broccoli tossed in oil
and lemon.

## FRIDAY

**Breakfast**
A ripe peach, a nectarine, or a bunch
of grapes.

**Light meal or snack**
Tossed green salad with plenty of
different salad leaves including, if
possible, rocket, oak leaves, and
lamb's lettuce and French Dressing
II (p.132).
Potato Galette (p.118).
Cauliflower steamed until just
*al dente* and tossed with a little
chopped parsley and butter.

**Main meal**
Tart Apple Slaw (p.73).
Fishburgers (p.93), with puréed
spinach and steamed carrots.

## SATURDAY

**Breakfast**
A feast of melon – try to have slices
of 2 or 3 different kinds.

**Light meal or snack**
Meze (p.78).
Thick Vegetable Soup with
Barley (p.79).
Rye crispbread with a little
cream cheese.

**Main meal**
Mixed green salad.
Tangerine Chicken Parcels (p.101).
Green beans and carrots.
Blackberry Parfait (p.155).

## SUNDAY

**Breakfast**
An orange.
Scrambled egg with grilled
mushrooms and tomatoes.

**Light meal or snack**
Salade Niçoise (p.70) – omit the
anchovy, and use only the yolk of the
hard-boiled egg.
Steamed broccoli tossed in a very
little butter.
A granary or wholewheat roll.
A ripe sweet pear.

**Main meal**
Avocado pears sliced and dressed
with a little oil, lemon juice, and
freshly ground pepper, served with
plenty of cress, on a bed of lettuce.
Pheasant with Apples, Celery,
and Cider (p.105).
Shredded cabbage cooked *al dente*.
Celery stalks with a selection of
different cheeses.
Grapes.

# WINTER

## MONDAY

### Breakfast
½ grapefruit.
An apple.
A serving of natural yogurt with a little honey and chopped nuts.

### Light meal or snack
Coleslaw II (p.128).
Baked potato with a little butter or 1tbs of sour cream and chopped fresh herbs.
A ripe sweet pear.

### Main meal
Fennel and Watercress Salad (p.131).
Gratin of Cauliflower and Broccoli (p.109).
A small piece of cheese, with sticks of celery.

## TUESDAY

### Breakfast
Porridge made with water, and 1tbs single cream.
1 slice wholewheat bread or toast with a little butter.

### Light meal or snack
Winter Salad (p.124).
A baked apple with sultanas, honey, and chopped walnuts.

### Main meal
Raw Artichoke Salad (p.122).
Grilled Spiced Chicken (p.100).
Steamed broccoli and carrots.

## WEDNESDAY

### Breakfast
Scrambled Eggs with Mushrooms (p.86).
A glass of orange juice.

### Light meal or snack
Lightly steamed cauliflower florets tossed in a little oil, and sprinkled with plenty of cress or finely chopped parsley.
Rice and Leek Minestrone (p.82).
A crusty wholewheat roll and butter.

### Main meal
Pepper and Onion Dip (p.143), together with sticks of celery, carrot, and fennel.
Rabbit with Black Olives (p.99).
Cauliflower and Artichoke Crush (p.114).

## THURSDAY

### Breakfast
Grapefruit juice.
Stewed apples sprinkled with some flaked almonds.
Natural yogurt.

### Light meal or snack
A tossed green salad.
Barley and Mushroom Casserole (p.133).
A ripe sweet pear.

### Main meal
Cabbage, Celery, and Apple Salad (p.126).
Aubergines Stuffed with Cheese (p.110).
Spinach purée.
Sticks of celery and an apple.

## FRIDAY

### Breakfast
Muesli (p.151), with a sliced banana, and a little single cream.

### Light meal or snack
Hot Beetroot Salad (p.129).
Black Olive Pâté (p.147), served on lettuce leaves with a crusty wholemeal roll and a little butter.
A ripe sweet pear.

### Main meal
Courgette, Garlic and Blue Cheese Soup (p.74).
Fish with a Spiced Yogurt Crust (p.96).
A big mixed salad.

## SATURDAY

### Breakfast
Dried Fruit Compôte (p.156), with 1tbs Greek yogurt.

### Light meal or snack
Watercress and Mushroom Salad (p.131).
Leek Pasties (p.148).
A banana.

### Main meal
½ grapefruit.
Omelette Arnold Bennett (p.88).
Green cabbage cooked al dente.
Tossed green salad.

## SUNDAY

### Breakfast
½ grapefruit.
2 rashers lean grilled bacon with a scrambled egg, mushrooms, and a grilled tomato.

### Light meal or snack
Sweetcorn Chowder (p.83).
Garlic Bread (p.151).
A mixed green salad with French Dressing II (p.132).

### Main meal
½ avocado with lemon juice and salt.
Sally's Lamb (p.106).
Red and Yellow Pepper Casserole (p.108).
Celery sticks and a selection of different cheeses.

# PACKED LUNCHES

Planning packed lunches that are either Starch or Protein is certainly trickier than making up a few sandwiches with cheese, salami, or cold chicken, adding a carton of yogurt, perhaps, and an apple. However, we hope the week of Starch and Protein packed lunches suggested here will prove that simple, varied, and delicious meals are actually quite easy to plan on the Superfoods Diet.

Delicatessens that cater to the lunchtime sandwich clientele in busy city centres often sell delicious mixed salads – as do most supermarkets. They also sell more obvious items like yogurt, cottage cheese, fresh fruit, packets of nuts, and dried fruit.

If you have time to make your own salads, save cottage cheese containers to store them in. The salads we suggest here will improve by being made a few hours ahead of the time they are eaten. In summer, when soft fruits are plentiful and cheap, you might buy some near your office, and have a refreshing fruit-only luncheon: strawberries are actually best eaten on their own. Add a pot of yogurt or cottage cheese if this sounds too insubstantial for you.

If you are cooking rice for dinner, make extra, add a dressing while it's still hot, and pack it for lunch the next morning, adding pieces of cucumber, tomato, black olives, cress, spring onions, or whatever salad stuffs you have in store.

In winter, make extra quantities of comforting, thick vegetable soups in the evening, and save some for next day's lunch. Heat it up in the morning, and transport it to work in the wide-mouthed thermos jars that general stores sell for schoolchildren.

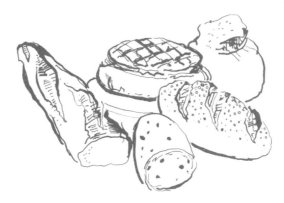

## PROTEIN PACKED LUNCHES

# MONDAY

A carton of natural cottage cheese.
An apple.
A hard-boiled egg.
Chunks of carrot, celery, cucumber, and fennel.

# TUESDAY

Cabbage, Celery, and Apple Salad (p.126).
An orange or a peach.
25g/1oz almonds, lightly roasted.
A pot of creamy yogurt.

# WEDNESDAY

Crudités with Tuna and Garlic Mayonnaise (p.144).
A carton of Stewed Apples with Ginger (p.155), with 2tbs yogurt stirred in.
Assorted nuts.

# THURSDAY

A piece of cold roast chicken or slices of cold roast turkey breast.
Apple, celery, and peanut salad.
A bunch of grapes.

# FRIDAY

A pot of natural yogurt.
Sticks of celery.
A piece of your favourite hard cheese.
An apple.

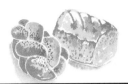

## STARCH PACKED LUNCHES

# MONDAY

Wholewheat pita pocket stuffed with slices of cucumber and tomato, sprigs of watercress, black olives, lettuce leaves, and a dribble of olive oil.
Raisins and nuts.

# TUESDAY

Wholewheat sandwiches with hard-boiled egg-yolks mashed with a little mayonnaise, slices of cucumber, and cress.
2 Dried Fruit Mini-Buns (p.157).
A banana.

# WEDNESDAY

A thermos jar of thick vegetable soup or minestrone.
A wholewheat roll or rye crackers with butter.
Grated carrot, onion, raisin, and hazelnut salad, with French Dressing II (p.132).

# THURSDAY

Rice salad.
Rye crispbread.
A ripe sweet pear.

# FRIDAY

Sticks of carrot, celery, fennel, cucumber, and sprigs of cauliflower, cleaned and packed in an airtight carton. A helping of ricotta cheese.
A crusty wholewheat roll with a little butter.

# FOR VEGETARIANS

A criticism often voiced of the diet made famous by Dr. Hay is that it could never work for vegetarians: they would have to live on beans and rice. In fact, vegetarians have a whole world of wonderful Superfoods to exploit when planning their menus. The fact that vegetarian meals need never be dull or unsatisfying is proved by the following sample week of glorious healthy eating.

Menus for a week from a lifetime of Harmonious Eating were supplied to us by Indian-born Keki Sidhwa, registered Naturopath and Osteopath, and President of the British Natural Hygiene Society, now retired.

"Nature Cure practitioners thought of Food Combining long before the Hay Diet was invented," says Keki, who has always encouraged his patients to try the regime. At mealtimes delicious smells waft from the Sidhwa kitchen. "I allow at least half an hour for eating," he says, "and half an hour afterwards in which to relax. I never read at mealtimes. I believe in doing one thing at a time. I am a gourmet. I like to be aware of what I am eating, and enjoy the taste of food."

In a typical week, here is how Keki Sidhwa eats.

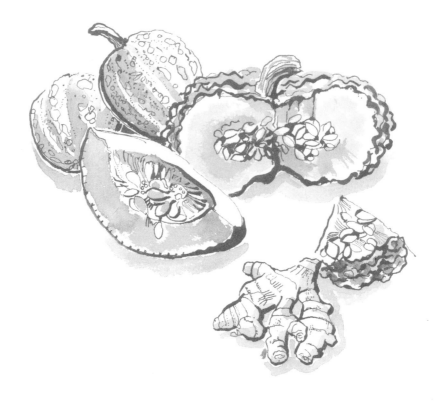

# A WEEK OF MENUS

## MONDAY

### Breakfast
½ pink grapefruit, 1 orange, 1 large apple, and 2 satsumas 25g/1oz almonds or sunflower or pumpkin seeds.

### Light meal or snack
Homemade thick vegetable broth (Thick Vegetable Soup with Barley on p.79) in winter or a glass of carrot juice; followed by a large vegetable salad and baked potatoes.

### Main meal
Side plate of green vegetable salad, cooked green vegetables, and stuffed peppers with lentils (Peppers Stuffed with Rice on p.134; substitute the same quantity of cooked lentils for the rice).

## TUESDAY

### Breakfast
2 ripe bananas, 1 pear, 250g/8oz of grapes, and 6 Hunza apricots.

### Light meal or snack
Keki's Lentil and Leek Soup (p.76) in winter or a glass of apple juice; followed by a large salad made with a variety of vegetables and 65g/2½oz nuts and seeds.

### Main meal
Side plate of salad, cooked green vegetables, and a Root Vegetable Casserole (p.119).

## WEDNESDAY

### Breakfast
2–3 thick slices of fresh pineapple, 1 kiwi fruit, 1 ripe mango, or 1 large apple. 125g/4oz live goat's milk yogurt, or Greek sheep's yogurt.

### Light meal or snack
Vegetable soup (try Springtime Minestrone on p.81), salad, and wholewheat bread and biscuits.

### Main meal
Salad, cooked green vegetables, and 2 poached eggs.

## THURSDAY

### Breakfast
125g/4oz crunchy oat cereal with 2tbs untreated fresh single cream.

### Light meal or snack
Bean soup (Beanfeast Broth on p.77) or a wineglass of apple or pineapple juice (125–150ml/4–6fl oz); vegetable salad, some low-fat soft cheese (50g/2oz), and 25g/1oz Edam, Cheddar, or Cheshire cheese.

### Main meal
Side plate of salad, cooked green and root vegetables, and some millet, or buckwheat, or brown rice.

## FRIDAY

### Breakfast
½ large melon.

### Light meal or snack
Soup or juice (carrot and celery), vegetable salad and brown rice savoury (Raw Vegetable Risotto on p.137).

### Main meal
Salad, cooked green vegetables, and butter beans, or bean stew of various beans (Full of Beans on p.112).

## SATURDAY

### Breakfast
A big tumbler of freshly juiced carrot and apple mixture or apple and orange juice mixture.

### Light meal or snack
Soup or juice, salad, and baked yams or sweet potatoes.

### Main meal
Salad. Cooked green vegetables, and Gratin of Cauliflower and Broccoli (p.109).

## SUNDAY

### Breakfast
A cup of hot water, plant milk and molasses, followed by 2 slices of wholewheat bread and butter.

### Light meal or snack
A large fruit plate of grapes, apple, pear, and ripe bananas, with some raisins and dates.

### Main meal
Salad, cooked green vegetables, and wholewheat macaroni or pasta (Pasta with Garlic, Oil, and Herb Sauce on p.139).

For those who would like to follow Keki's menu, we have included two of his specialities in our Recipe section – Keki's Leek and Lentil Soup, and Root Vegetable Casserole. Elsewhere, suggestions for similar dishes from our Recipes will be found in brackets.

# SPECIAL OCCASIONS

Birthday and anniversary celebrations, Christmas and Thanksgiving feasts, dinner parties and family get-togethers are the downfall of most diets. Our suggested menus for Special Occasions prove that the Superfoods Diet meets every challenge.

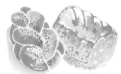

## PROTEIN MEALS

### SPRING

Watercress Soup (p.70).
Salmon with Orange Sauce (p.91).
Young peas and broad beans.
Tossed Green Salad (p.121).
Cheese, celery, and nuts.

### SUMMER

Courgette, Garlic and Blue Cheese Soup (p.74).
Cold Chicken Rothschild with Grapes, served with Lemon and Tarragon Sauce (p.101).
Red and Yellow Pepper Casserole (p.108).
Fennel and Watercress Salad (p.131).
Gooseberry and Elderflower Fool (p.153).

### AUTUMN

Gazpacho (p.71).
Curried Chicken with Peaches (p.102).
Cauliflower and Artichoke Crush (p.114).
Watercress salad.
Peaches in White Wine with Preserved Ginger (p.155).

### WINTER

Beetroot and Apple Soup (p.72).
Pheasant with Apple, Celery, and Cider (p.105).
Steamed broccoli.
Creamed Onions (p.114).
Stewed Apples with Ginger (p.155): (serve in individual glass bowls, topped with Greek yogurt, and pieces of preserved ginger).

## STARCH MEALS

### SPRING

Springtime Minestrone (p.81), with hot, crusty rolls.
Onion Quiche (p.147).
Green Beans with Garlic and Chilli (p.113).
Tossed Green Salad (p.121) with French Dressing II (p.132).
Sliced sweet pears with cream and raisins.

### SUMMER

Almond and Carrot Cream (p.78).
Raw Vegetable Risotto (p.137).
Cucumber and Watercress Salad (p.131).
Tropical Fruit Salad (p.157).

### AUTUMN

Meze (p.78), with hot *pita* bread.
Angela's Spiced Chickpea Casserole (p.138).
Red Radicchio and Chicory Salad (p.130).
Spiced Rice Cream (p.156).

### WINTER

Jerusalem Artichoke Cream (p.79).
Pasta with Red Pepper Sauce (p.140).
Tossed green salad with watercress and rocket.
Baked Bananas (p.157).

CHAPTER 7

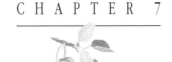

# INTENSIVE WEIGHT LOSS

We are absolutely opposed to any form of crash-dieting — not just because it's extremely unhealthy and can even be dangerous, but also because it is almost invariably counter-productive, too. Lost kilos pile back on again within weeks or even days of you losing weight. Even to readers who are seriously overweight, we strongly recommend that you try the Superfoods Diet as outlined above, without attempting to modify it any further by obsessive calorie-counting. We are certain that if you follow it carefully, you will soon begin to notice a slow but steady loss of weight. Furthermore, because it is such a simple and enjoyable diet, you will be able to stay with it until you reach your ideal weight — by which time Harmonious Eating will be a way of life for you.

If, however, you have serious medical reasons — or pressing personal ones — for losing a lot of excess weight as soon as possible, you may like to try our Intensive Weight Loss plan. It's a streamlined, lighter form of the Superfoods Diet, which will still allow you to enjoy meal-times. We suggest you try it for one week ONLY initially.

You will certainly find this regime easier to stick with than most ordinary diets. You may even decide to stay with it for several weeks, until you have reached your target weight. If you find it tough going, don't give up altogether and go on a despairing binge, just revert to the ordinary Superfoods Diet from the next mealtime. There are a number of simple rules for the Intensive Weight Loss plan. To make it even easier, we've worked out four weeks of menus for you: for spring, summer, autumn, and winter.

**Try the Intensive Weight Loss plan for one week**

## THE RULES

● Follow the basic Rules of the Superfoods Diet.

● You may include any of the recipes in the Recipes section, except those marked with a star ★.

● Omit the following foods from your diet: roast beef, roast lamb, roast pork, and roast chicken and roast duck served with its skin. Any combination of meat and cheese. Double, clotted, and whipped cream. Fried and scrambled eggs. High-fat cheeses like Gruyère, mature Cheddar, Gorgonzola, and Stilton. Sauces made with cheese. Butter in lavish amounts – although you can eat a little with your toast or roll.

● Avoid made-up or processed foods, particularly those containing sugar in any form, or high amounts of fat.

● Don't drink alcohol – and certainly not spirits. If you find this tough, relax the rules just at weekends. On Saturday and Sunday, allow yourself EITHER one glass of beer or lager with a Starch meal, OR one glass of good wine with a Protein meal.

● Substitute low-fat yogurt for Greek yogurt, and low-fat cottage cheese for regular cottage cheese. And have skimmed or partially skimmed milk in your tea or coffee.

● For salads, use just 1–2 tsp of the appropriate dressing.

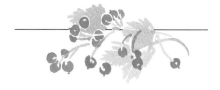

# SPRING

## MONDAY

**Breakfast**
Cold Spiced Apricots (p.153).
2tbs low-fat yogurt.

**Light meal or snack**
A big mixed salad – radishes, spring
onions, celery, grated carrots,
cucumber, red and yellow peppers,
sliced cabbage, young dandelion
leaves, lettuce, mint, and parsley.
Low-fat cottage cheese.
An apple.

**Main meal**
Raw Vegetable Risotto (p.137).
Green Beans with Garlic and
Chilli (p.113).

## TUESDAY

**Breakfast**
A large ripe pear, sliced, with 2tbs
single cream and a few raisins.

**Light meal or snack**
Tossed Green Salad (p.121), with
grated carrots.
Pasta with Piquant Red Sauce (p.140).

**Main meal**
Watercress Soup (p.70).
Poached trout with a squeeze
of lemon juice.
Puréed spinach.
Lightly steamed baby carrots.

## WEDNESDAY

**Breakfast**
Low-fat yogurt with honey, a
squeeze of orange, chopped nuts,
and a dusting of cinnamon.

**Light meal or snack**
Sticks of carrot, celery, and fennel.
Springtime Minestrone (p.81).
Courgettes tossed in a little oil.

**Main meal**
Red Radicchio, Iceberg Lettuce,
and Rocket Salad (p.124).
Turkey Breast with Lemon and
White Wine (p.105).
Spring greens.

## THURSDAY

**Breakfast**
An apple.
A pear.
A helping of low-fat yogurt.

**Light meal or snack**
Easy Mackerel Dip (p.142), with a
big platter of raw vegetables – sticks
of carrot, fennel, celery, red and
yellow peppers, baby courgettes,
radishes, and spring onions.

**Main meal**
Cucumber and Watercress
Salad (p.131).
Sicilian Pasta with Fennel (p.141).

## FRIDAY

**Breakfast**
Dried Fruit Compôte (p.156).

**Light meal or snack**
Tossed Green Salad (p.121), with
French Dressing II (p.132), and a
plateful of young spring vegetables:
baby carrots, courgettes, turnips,
new potatoes, and peas, all steamed
until just *al dente*, and tossed with a
nut of butter, and plenty of chopped
parsley and mint.

**Main meal**
Apple and Watercress Soup (p.72).
Cold Poached Fish (p.94 ) with
Fresh Tomato Sauce (p.95).
Green beans.

## SATURDAY

**Breakfast**
An apple.
A pear.
A helping of low-fat natural yogurt.

**Light meal or snack**
Stuffed Pita Pockets (p.149).

**Main meal**
Avocado, Spinach, and Mushroom
Salad (p.122).
Grilled Spiced Chicken (p.100).
Steamed baby carrots and turnips.

## SUNDAY

**Breakfast**
A feast of fresh fruit in season.

**Light meal or snack**
Tossed Green Salad (p.121) with
French Dressing II (p.132).
Baked Eggs with Spinach and
Mushrooms (p.89).

**Main meal**
Lettuce and watercress salad.
Rabbit with Anchovy Sauce (p.98).
Steamed carrots and green beans.
Spiced Apricots (p.153). (Make
enough for 2 meals.)

# SUMMER

## MONDAY

### Breakfast
½ grapefruit.
A poached or boiled egg with 2 grilled tomatoes.

### Light meal or snack
Avocado, Tomato, and Mushroom Salad (p.126).
A helping of low-fat cottage cheese.
A bunch of grapes.

### Main meal
Cucumber Salad (p.130).
Stir-fried Vegetables with Rice (p.136).

## TUESDAY

### Breakfast
A sliced peach with 4 or 5 strawberries.

### Light meal or snack
A green salad, and a plateful of new season's vegetables: baby carrots, courgettes, turnips, new potatoes, peas, all steamed until just *al dente*, then tossed with a nut of butter, and plenty of chopped parsley and mint.

### Main meal
Gazpacho (p.71).
Stuffed Courgettes (p.108), with carrots and spinach.

## WEDNESDAY

### Breakfast
A bowl of cherries.

### Light meal or snack
Tossed Green Salad (p.121), with French Dressing II (p.132).
Pasta with Garlic, Oil, and Herb Sauce (p.139).

### Main meal
Sliced cucumber salad with a dressing of 1tbs yogurt, 1tsp of oil, seasoning, a little chopped garlic, and plenty of fresh chopped mint.
Curried Chicken with Peaches (p.102), with quartered lemons and tomatoes, and chunks of iceberg lettuce.

## THURSDAY

### Breakfast
A peach and a nectarine.

### Light meal or snack
Lettuce and rocket salad.
Low-fat cottage cheese with chunks of cucumber and tomato.
Steamed courgettes.

### Main meal
Broad Bean and Mushroom Salad (p.128).
Aubergine and Onion Pilaff (p.135).
A slice of wholewheat bread or a crusty wholewheat roll.
Spinach purée.

## FRIDAY

### Breakfast
A big bunch of grapes.

### Light meal or snack
Millet Croquettes (p.149), with Fresh Tomato Sauce (p.94).
Tiny new courgettes steamed and tossed with a little butter and chopped parsley.

### Main meal
Spinach and watercress salad.
Onion and Garlic Soup (p.75).
Cold Poached Fish (p.94) with Lemon and Yogurt Sauce (p.95).
Runner beans.

## SATURDAY

### Breakfast
A feast of summer fruit: a peach, a ripe apricot, some grapes, and a nectarine.

### Light meal or snack
A big mixed salad. Include any of the following – tomatoes, cucumber, rocket, skinned raw broad beans, sorrel or young dandelion leaves, and any kind of lettuce, with French Dressing II (p.132). A plate of steamed baby new potatoes, tossed in a nut of butter with plenty of finely chopped mint.

### Main meal
Prawns with Pink Grapefruit (p.75) served on a bed of iceberg lettuce and watercress.
Courgette Frittata (p.84).
French beans and sliced carrots.

## SUNDAY

### Breakfast
A hot crusty roll with a little butter.

### Light meal or snack
Fruit and Cottage Cheese Salad (p.123) – use low-fat cottage cheese.
A peach.

### Main meal
Borscht (p.76).
Welsh Salt Duck (p.103), with an orange and watercress salad.
Mangetout peas.

# AUTUMN

## MONDAY

### Breakfast
$\frac{1}{2}$ grapefruit.
A soft-boiled egg with a grilled tomato.

### Light meal or snack
Tossed Green Salad (p.121).
Tomatoes Stuffed with Cottage Cheese and Tuna (p.142) – use low-fat cottage cheese.

### Main meal
Red Salad (p.130).
Vegetable Curry (p.117).
A wholewheat roll or slice of bread.

## TUESDAY

### Breakfast
A big bunch of grapes.

### Light meal or snack
Red Radicchio and Chicory Salad (p.130).
Mushrooms Provençale (p.119) with a crusty wholemeal roll or granary roll.
A ripe sweet pear.

### Main meal
Cabbage, Celery, and Apple Salad (p.126).
Grilled trout with quarters of lemon and tomatoes.
Steamed or lightly boiled cauliflower florets, tossed in a little oil and lemon, and garnished with plenty of chopped parsley.

## WEDNESDAY

### Breakfast
A peach and a nectarine.

### Light meal or snack
Lettuce and grated carrot salad.
Baked potato with Fresh Tomato Sauce (p.95).
Steamed courgettes.

### Main meal
$\frac{1}{2}$ avocado with lemon juice and a little seasoning.
Grilled Spiced Chicken (p.100), with chunks of lemon, cucumber, tomato, and iceberg lettuce.

## THURSDAY

### Breakfast
Sliced oranges and pink grapefruit with a helping of low-fat yogurt.

### Light meal or snack
2 hard-boiled eggs with a helping of low-fat cottage cheese, and chunks of tomato, cucumber, and fennel, with 2tsp of olive oil and a little seasoning

### Main meal
Fennel and Watercress Salad (p.131).
Macrobiotic Millet (p.134).
Green cabbage sliced and steam-cooked in a covered pan for no more than a couple of minutes – it should be green and crunchy when you serve it.

## FRIDAY

### Breakfast
Blackberries, low-fat yogurt, and 1tsp of honey.

### Light meal or snack
Tossed Green Salad (p.121), with French Dressing II (p.132).
Pasta with Cauliflower and Broccoli Sauce (p.141).
A wholewheat roll or a slice of wholewheat bread.

### Main meal
Crudités (p.142).
Grilled fillets of whiting with a small nut of butter, and plenty of finely chopped herbs.
Braised fennel.

## SATURDAY

### Breakfast
A big bunch of grapes.

### Light meal or snack
Black olives, radishes, sticks of carrot, and fennel.
Rice, Artichoke, and Potato Minestrone (p.82).
A wholewheat roll.
A ripe sweet pear or a banana.

### Main meal
Beetroot and Apple Soup (p.72).
Rabbit with Black Olives (p.99), with Cauliflower and Artichoke Crush (p.114).

## SUNDAY

### Breakfast
Dried Fruit Compôte (p.156), with 1tsp of single cream.

### Light meal or snack
Tossed Green Salad (p.121), with French Dressing II (p.132).
Black Olive Pâté (p.147), with crusty wholemeal bread.
A plateful of steamed vegetables: slices of carrot, cauliflower florets, and chunks of fennel.

### Main meal
Nectarine and Pink Grapefruit Salad with Sour Cream Dressing (p.68).
Turkey with Anchovy Sauce (p.104).
Steamed broccoli.
Sticks of celery and low-fat cheese.

# WINTER

## MONDAY

### Breakfast
Porridge made with water, and eaten with 2tsp of single cream, and a little honey.

### Light meal or snack
Fruit and Cottage Cheese Salad (p.123) – use low-fat cottage cheese.

### Main meal
Watercress and Mushroom Salad (p.131).
Stir-fried Vegetables with Rice (p.136).

## TUESDAY

### Breakfast
Stewed apples with low-fat yogurt.

### Light meal or snack
Sticks of carrot, celery, and fennel.
Thick Vegetable Soup with Barley (p.79).
A wholewheat roll or a slice of wholewheat bread.
A plateful of green cabbage tossed with a little butter, and seasoned with nutmeg.

### Main meal
½ avocado with lemon juice and a little seasoning.
Cold Poached Fish (p.94) with Fresh Tomato Sauce (p.95).
Green or white cabbage cooked until *al dente*.

## WEDNESDAY

### Breakfast
A bowl of orange, grapefruit, and tangerine segments.

### Light meal or snack
Fennel and Watercress Salad (p.131).
Pasta with Red Pepper Sauce (p.140).

### Main meal
Raw Artichoke Salad (p.122).
Grilled chicken breast with grilled red and yellow peppers, dressed with 1tsp of olive oil and a little lemon.
Steamed florets of cauliflower and broccoli, tossed with a little nutmeg and butter.

## THURSDAY

### Breakfast
Greek yogurt with a little honey and a few chopped almonds.

### Light meal or snack
Coleslaw I (p.124) – make a big one.
An apple.

### Main meal
Meze (p.78).
Angela's Spiced Chickpea Casserole (p.138).
*Pita* bread.
A green salad.

## FRIDAY

### Breakfast
A sliced apple and a sliced pear, with a few sesame seeds.

### Light meal or snack
Spinach and lettuce salad with plenty of fresh chopped herbs.
Millet Croquettes (p.149), with Creamed Onions (p.114).

### Main meal
Radicchio, Iceberg Lettuce, and Rocket Salad (p.124).
Fresh grilled trout with a squeeze of lemon juice.
Cauliflower and Artichoke Crush (p.114).

## SATURDAY

### Breakfast
A banana sliced with a few raisins, and 1tsp of single cream.

### Light meal or snack
Crudités (p.142).
Rice and Leek Minestrone (p.82).
A wholewheat roll or a stick of granary bread with a little butter.

### Main meal
½ grapefruit.
A 2-egg omelette made with plenty of chopped fresh herbs.
Brussels Sprouts Gratin (p.111).
A green salad.
Sticks of celery, and a little low-fat cream cheese or cottage cheese.

## SUNDAY

### Breakfast
A hot, crusty wholewheat roll with a little butter.

### Light meal or snack
Salad of iceberg lettuce, with plenty of cress, grated carrots, celery, spring onions, sunflower seeds, and raisins, with French Dressing II (p.132).
A baked potato with a little low-fat cottage cheese.
A ripe sweet pear.

### Main meal
Steamed globe artichokes with a dip made from 1tsp of low-fat yogurt, 1tsp of olive oil, and 1tsp of lemon juice seasoned to taste.
Stir-fried Turkey Breasts with Celery, Walnuts, and Oranges (p.104).
Steamed broccoli.
A baked apple stuffed with raisins, almonds, and a little honey.

CHAPTER 8

# THE SUPERFOODS

Rule One of the Superfoods Diet is: Eat Superfoods. Here are profiles of the most important ones – wonder-working foods that build health and vitality, foods that nourish your brain and your nervous system as well as skin, bones, muscles, veins, and arteries. Eat Superfoods with their rainbow spectrum of nutrients, and you will ensure that the appestat mechanism in your mid-brain works efficiently to help maintain you at a reasonable weight and in good shape. Eat Superfoods and enjoy them: they are Nature's own best diet.

**Almonds** are a highly concentrated food, which we should all enjoy more often. They are rich in protein – they are actually 20 per cent protein – in essential fatty acids, and in some of the vital B vitamins. They are also good sources of important minerals – zinc, magnesium, potassium, and iron. Eat vitamin C-rich foods at the same time, though, since almonds also contain oxalic and phytic acid, which can prevent your absorption of these minerals.

Half a dozen almonds can turn a light snack into a well-balanced meal. Almonds with their rich blandness make the basis of delicious soups. On the Superfoods Diet, ground almonds can replace starchy thickeners in gravy or sauces. You can use them as a topping – instead of conventional high-fat, high-starch crumbles – for fruit puddings, on special occasions when

you feel you deserve a treat. Try our Peach Pudding on p.154.

**Apples** We all know what an apple a day does to your doctor's income. So what's in an apple? A bonus for your heart: the pectin and vitamin C in apples help keep cholesterol levels stable, as American studies have shown, and counter the ravages of pollution. The malic and tartaric acids in apples help neutralize the acid by-products of indigestion, and help your body cope with excess protein or rich, fatty foods. Apple purée with pork, apples with cheese, or sage and apple stuffing for goose are gourmet recipes based on country wisdom.

Baked apples are a wholesome treat every child enjoys: serve them stuffed with raisins, with ground almonds, or with blackberries when they are in season. Enjoy rich Greek yogurt with them instead of custard

or cream. When apples are cheap and plentiful, make quantities of purée. Sweeten with a little honey, spiked in winter with all the heartwarming, digestive spices, such as nutmeg, cinnamon, and cloves, in summer, sharpen the purée with refreshing lemon juice. Try a raw apple purée: it needs to be made fast, before the sliced apples turn brown. Have half a cupful of lemon juice or pineapple juice sitting in your food processor as you feed apple slices in. Stirred into plain yogurt, eaten with a few nuts, puréed apple could be a perfect start to the day.

**Apricots** are loaded with beta-carotene, the natural precursor of vitamin A, as their wonderful yellow-orange colour informs us – the brighter the fruit, the more beta-carotene there is. Plump, sun-ripened, fresh fruit is a treat best enjoyed in the Mediterranean, where apricots are locally grown. Dried apricots are a year-round treat. The best way to enjoy them is simply well-washed, then put in a basin with boiling water poured over them, and left to plump at their leisure. For a more sophisticated version, try Spiced Apricots (see p.153).

**Artichokes, globe,** are the friend of the liver, as any Frenchman will tell you, and extracts from this vegetable feature prominently – as do those of the dandelion – in bitter alcoholic drinks intended to stimulate the appetite, or soothe the troubled liver after an evening's excesses at the dinner-table or bar.

Artichokes need to be perfectly fresh: the globes should be firm, with the leaves tightly packed together. Don't buy them if they look wilted or dry. Italians are also gluttons for artichokes, and market stalls groan with their weight, complete with long stems and trailing leaves. Tender young artichokes are often eaten raw, with a little grated parmesan and an olive oil and lemon dressing, when their taste is fresh and piquant. Cooked, they feature in a dozen pasta or risotto recipes, braised with broad beans – a lovely combination – or in soups like Rice, Artichoke, and Potato Minestrone on p.82. Trimmed, cooked, and cold, they feature on every restaurant menu, dressed with a little oil and parsley.

To prepare artichokes for eating in any of these ways, have a chunk of lemon to hand ready for rubbing the cut bits – otherwise they will discolour – and a pan of water with a dash of vinegar into which you will throw the prepared artichokes. Choose small, tender ones, and cut the stems off under the leaves. Remove any old, dry, or wilted outer leaves, then with a sharp knife pare off the tips of the leaves neatly.

**Artichokes, Jerusalem** The chore of preparing these knobbly little vegetables has been eased in recent years by the introduction of a purpose-bred, smoother, rounder variety. Either way, we think they're a ridiculously underestimated gourmet treat, with a lovely smoky flavour. Use them for delicious winter soups, or for a purée that is especially delicious with chicken or any form of game. They are high in potassium, especially useful in today's typical high-salt diet.

**Asparagus** is another gourmet treat that actually benefits the liver – and the kidneys too, of which its active compound, asparagine, is a stimulant. During its brief season it does seem almost criminal to eat asparagus in any way other than the simplest – steamed, hot, with melted butter, or cold with mayonnaise. Leave plenty of stalk on them unless the stems are very tough and woody.

**Avocado pears** Every slimmer knows that luscious avocado pears are a high-fat, high-calorie treat. But they are also almost a complete food, supplying a little protein and starch as well as the pure oil that is mainly a mono-unsaturated fat. Avocados are also potassium-rich, and a good source of vitamin A; they supply some B complex, a little vitamin C, and even vitamin E. So we certainly recommend that you enjoy them as part of the basic Superfoods Diet.

In our view, the best way to enjoy them is the simplest. Eat them with the juice from a chunk of fresh lemon, a little salt, and freshly ground pepper. Elaborate dressings – or piles of woolly shrimps coated in pink sauce – can destroy their delicious but delicate flavour.

Avocados, incidentally, are often thought of as a dangerously "rich" food: in fact, the fats they contain are particularly easy to digest.

**Bananas,** one of Nature's most popular Fast Foods, are often unjustly maligned as a high-calorie snack. In fact, the average banana contains under 100 calories, and is packed with nourishment – particularly potassium, which is essential to the functioning of every single cell in our bodies. Zinc, iron, folic acid, and calcium are other goodies, plus a lot of that useful fibre, pectin. Bananas – as long as they are ripe – are a wonderfood for

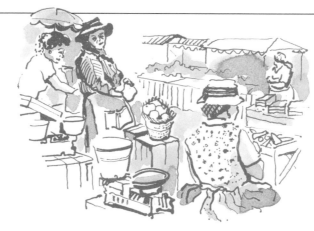

**Eat fresh, locally grown Superfoods in season for good value, flavour, and nutrition**

the digestive tract, soothing and helping to normalize function. Bananas are particularly welcome to Superfoods Dieters since their bland sweetness makes them one of the rare fruits that can be enjoyed with a Starch meal.

**Barley,** like other grains, is mineral-rich, with particularly high levels of calcium and potassium, and plenty of B-complex vitamins, making it useful for people suffering from stress or fatigue. Recent research has shown that barley is also endowed with remarkable cholesterol-lowering powers; and in traditional medicine it has always been prized for its soothing, demulcent qualities. So there are good reasons to enjoy this rather neglected grain more often than we do.

Nutritionally, pot barley – the little, beige, dehulled grain – is superior to cleaned or pearl barley, as well as having much more flavour. Enjoy it in warming and comforting dishes for a cold winter's day: a tablespoon of barley added to any simple vegetable soup will turn it into a satisfying meal.

**Beans** Fresh green beans – either the thin, rounded pods or else those flat, pale ones – are one of the great treats of early summer. Their freshness is vital: we can't understand why people pay fortunes outside their season for beans grown in exotic places and transported thousands of miles to our supermarkets. When green beans are young and fresh, they are at their best simply boiled until just cooked through, and then served with a little oil or butter. Broad beans can be eaten raw when small and young – slip them out of their rather indigestible skins first. The herb summer savory might have been invented to accompany beans: it improves their digestibility – which has always been under a faint cloud – while enhancing their flavour.

**Beef and lamb (from biologically reared livestock)** Growing public demand ensures that supermarkets now stock these healthier meats. Beef and lamb produced this way are much lower in fat than meat from intensively reared livestock – which can contain up to 30 per cent fat, most of it highly saturated. They are also free from the cocktail of chemicals with which most beef and lamb are normally laced – hormones, growth accelerators, and the accumulated residue of pesticides to which the livestock has certainly been exposed.

Beef and lamb free of these nasties – and of resulting problems such as BSE – are good sources of protein, of two vital minerals, iron and zinc, and of many B-complex vitamins. On the Superfoods Diet, red meat should be an occasional treat rather than a regular item, to be eaten no more than once or twice a week.

**Beetroot** In Romany medicine, beetroot juice was used as a blood-builder, for patients who were pale and run-down. In Russia and Eastern Europe, it is used both to build up resistance, and to treat convalescents after a serious illness. In fact, fresh raw beet juice is a powerful blood-cleanser and tonic, which has also been valued for centuries for its usefulness to the digestive system generally, and to the liver in particular – except when, as so often, drenched in hyperacid vinegars.

These powers are certainly enhanced when the beetroot is eaten raw. The popular French starter *crudités* – literally, raw foods – which combines grated raw beetroot, raw carrot, and perhaps paper-thin slices of cucumber, all dressed with olive oil and lemon juice, and garnished with chopped parsley – is a more powerful tonic for general health than a whole bottle of vitamin pills. The limp, flabby pre-cooked

beetroot you find in the corner greengrocer doesn't seem to us worth buying. If you've never eaten it raw and enjoyed its tart, earthy taste, you're missing a treat. Look for uncooked beetroot, wash and pare off the skin, and grate it raw for a salad. Pile it on top of cottage cheese, perhaps. Try it in an uncooked summer soup, too – see Beetroot and Apple Soup on p.72. For an unusual hot vegetable dish, try softening a little finely chopped onion in butter in a small pan, grating the beetroot straight in on top of it. Then add a dash of lemon juice, or a spoonful of cream and a sprinkling of parsley.

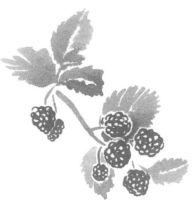

**Blackberries** are best gathered wild, well away from the lead pollution of passing cars, or the attentions of zealous pesticide-sprayers. Wash them and enjoy them raw: they supply not only vitamin C but also – unusually for a fruit – a lot of vitamin E, too. (There's much less vitamin E in those big, rather tasteless, cultivated ones, though.) Cooked, they combine particularly well with apples.

**Blackcurrants** are rich in vitamin C in a highly stable form, and other mysterious health-giving properties of this fruit have been honoured for centuries in country medicine. Blackcurrants picked and eaten straight off the bush, with the sun still warm on them, are a gourmet treat, and they are at their best eaten raw. Combine them with raspberries, the last of the strawberries, and some bilberries – if you can find them – for a wonderful summer treat: redcurrants and raspberries are a classic combination.

**Broccoli** comes in two varieties: the long, green stems, or the smaller, denser, bluish-purplish kind, like miniature cauliflowers. It belongs to the mighty crucifer family, whose protective powers against cancer have been demonstrated in a number of studies. Other crucifers include cabbage, cauliflower, kale, radishes, horseradish, spring greens, turnips, and brussels sprouts.

Broccoli is also rich in iron, in vitamin C (while raw or only lightly cooked), in beta-carotene, the plant precursor of vitamin A, and in folic acid. So the fresher and greener you eat it, the better. And, in fact, when it is steam-cooked until just *al dente*, it can be eaten and enjoyed like asparagus, with nothing more than a little butter for accompaniment. Eat the carefully washed heads of uncooked broccoli – as long as they are crisp and fresh – with a savoury dip: there are several to choose from on pp.142–4. Like cauliflower, broccoli also lends itself to gratin dishes (see p.109, for an example).

**Cabbage** This inexpensive vegetable has probably been the subject of more serious medical research than

any other foodstuff. Its remarkable healing powers – long attested in traditional medicine, and now being demonstrated in laboratories and hospitals – cover a startling range of ailments, including respiratory infections, cancer, and heart disease.

Most of these therapeutic effects have been observed with raw cabbage, and no doubt would be found also in sauerkraut. The long, dismal stewing cabbage sometimes undergoes in cookery not only deactivates much of this healing potential, but also ruins it for the palate, and makes it indigestible. Cook it like spinach: well washed and shredded, in a tightly sealed pan, over a low heat, in no more than a tablespoon or two of water, and *please,* no salt. After two or three minutes it will be fresh, crunchy, bright green, and utterly delicious. Add a knob of butter and a dusting of nutmeg, or a trickle of oil and lemon juice.

Shredded white cabbage makes good salads, combining well with nuts or apples (try Tart Apple Slaw on p.73), and forming the basis of popular coleslaw. Cut away the thick central stalks and ribs. For a salad with real crunch, try combining shredded white cabbage with celery and apple, and marinating it for a couple of hours in pineapple juice.

**Carrots** are another of the great Superfoods, so rich in beta-carotene that a single carrot will supply your

vitamin A needs for an entire day. Eating carrots will up levels of red blood cells, and studies have also shown that carrots have a protective action against excess ultra-violet or radiation. So if you want to stay young, healthy, and free from wrinkles, you should include plenty of carrots in your diet.

Get into the excellent habit of scraping a couple of fresh carrots and cutting them into fingers, for you and your family to nibble at the start of a meal. Preparation takes seconds – and the result does wonders for your digestion as well as your general health.

Carrots have a thousand uses in cooking: in soups, in stews, in salads, and as a principal ingredient in *crudités* (see p.142). One of the best soups we know, a great party piece, combines the glowing colours of carrot and orange: try our variation adding ginger, on p.73.

**Celeriac,** the root of celery, is slowly becoming more popular. Try it in the French *céleri rémoulade*: peeled, cut into strips, blanched for a couple of minutes, then dressed with a mayonnaise into which you have stirred plenty of mustard, and left to marinate in this for a while.

Celeriac is also delicious cooked, when its slightly smoky flavour becomes more pronounced. Try celeriac in a purée combined with potatoes (see p.116).

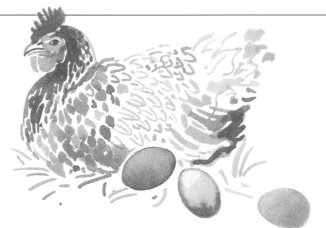

**Free-range eggs and chickens supply first-class protein**

**Celery** helps calm the nerves, according to Hippocrates – perhaps because of its rich calcium content. Its strong effect on the kidneys helps to eliminate wastes via the urine. And worldwide, it has a high reputation as an antirheumatic.

Celery is so delicious raw, as long as it is still fresh, crisp, and crunchy, that it hardly seems worth cooking. The braised celery served up in many restaurants – limp, grey, and watery – is enough to put one off the idea. Instead, enjoy celery as the perfect accompaniment to cheese, or eaten in sticks, along with carrots and cucumber, as the simplest of starters to a meal, or in a mixed salad.

Never throw away the leaves and trimmings of celery – boil them up to make a wonderful stock!

**Chicken, free-range,** not only tastes vastly superior to the flabby battery hen (which occasionally has an odour of fish) it is also lower in saturated fat, and free of many of the dubious chemicals, including stress chemicals, poured into battery birds during their brief, unhappy lifespans. Chicken is lower in fat than red meat, and most of the fat is in the skin, and thus easily removed.

**Chicory** is one of a family of winter salad vegetables (other members are the endives), all of which are related to wild chicory. This plant has always had a powerful reputation in traditional medicine as a cleanser

and detoxifier, one of the great spring tonics. The yellow-tipped white cones that we call chicory – and the French, confusingly, *endives* – are a welcome addition to the salad range in winter. They are firm enough to combine well with soft, fruity textures like oranges or avocados, or with a sharp lemony dressing. Cooked, chicory loses its looks – but develops a pleasant, slightly bitter flavour.

**Dandelion** You won't find dandelion leaves at your greengrocer or supermarket, but if you have a garden, cultivate a patch of this attractive, yellow-flowered weed – or harvest them, well away from roads or drift from agricultural spraying, on walks in the country.

The bitter taste of dandelion leaves is a clue to their usefulness and, in fact, they have a centuries-long reputation in the treatment of liver and digestive problems. They are rich in vitamin A and vitamin C, and they have more iron than spinach. In France they star in a well-known salad, in which they are tossed with bits of frizzled bacon in a mild olive oil. Add the young leaves – the older leaves are too bitter – to any mixed green salad, to soups, to the pan with spinach, or to make vegetable stocks.

**Dates,** like figs, are a highly energizing and nourishing foodstuff. Bedouin Arabs travel for days across

the desert with little more than a few dates, figs, and a little meal by way of food. In the Superfoods Diet, both dates and figs are permitted fruits with Starch meals – an agreeable end to a meal to those with an intractable sweet tooth. In her *Fruit Book*, Jane Grigson warns, however, that dates should be split open and the stones removed before eating. Make sure they are free of insect infestation. She points out that dates are often dusted with toxic preservatives, and then coated with glycerine to give them that attractive stickiness. Fresh dates imported from Israel are probably the healthiest buy. (It's always productive to write to the manager of your local supermarket questioning treatment methods of this kind: evidence of customer concern has prompted most of the major advances in healthy eating now possible in Britain.)

As energy food, put three or four dates in a Starch-packed lunch to replace that bar of chocolate.

**Eggs, free-range**, like the birds that lay them, are also free of factory-farming chemicals. Eggs supply first-class protein, zinc, and B vitamins, as well as other nutrients.

**Game** is free-range by definition, and thus – like meat from biologically reared livestock – free of many of the chemicals found in factory-farmed meat. Thanks to

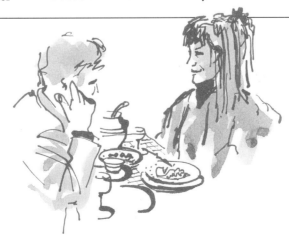

their highly active lifestyle, game-birds are also much lower in saturated fat than beef or lamb – fat is around 4 per cent of their total body weight, no more – and they supply plenty of iron.

**Garlic** enjoys a high double reputation: as a mainstay of Mediterranean cuisine, and as the king of all healing plants. No other plant has enjoyed such a high reputation – in so many different countries and civilizations – for helping such a wide range of ailments, particularly in the degenerative diseases such as cancer, heart problems, premature ageing, and major infectious diseases. Eat garlic regularly, and you will not only enhance your cooking: you'll be doing your health a favour, too.

Add garlic to soups, stews, fish, and meat dishes – even the most pallid and boring of chickens takes on appeal when anointed with olive oil, crushed garlic, and *herbes de provence*. Eat garlic chopped raw in salads – none of this puritan mere-rub-around-the-salad-bowl nonsense, please. Eat it in marvellous golden *aioli* – mayonnaise, which incorporates two or three cloves of garlic. Cold chicken or plain, poached white fish, served hot with *aioli* on the side, is a dish fit for a king. So are plain boiled potatoes. One of the simplest of all snacks is Garlic Bread (see p.151) – children always love it.

**Grapefruit,** like other citrus fruit, is rich in vitamin C and the fibre pectin, as well as in bioflavonoids, which recent studies have shown to enhance the effect of vitamin C. Bioflavonoids in citrus fruit are found in the segment skins and the pith, so eat the whole fruit rather than just the juice.

**Grapes** are the present that kind people take to their sick friends: nothing could be better for them. Grapes are a uniquely nourishing, strengthening, cleansing, and regenerating food, useful for convalescents, for the anemic, and for those suffering from stress, depression, or fatigue.

Start a meal, if you like, with a bunch of grapes; but don't end one with grapes, since they, like melon, ferment rapidly in the stomach. There's really only one way to eat and enjoy grapes: well washed, on their own, and as they come.

**Kiwifruit** are loaded with nutritional wealth – almost twice as much vitamin C as oranges, more fibre than an apple, and as much vitamin E as an avocado. They are particularly rich in potassium (of which Western diets, high in sodium from processed foods, can be dangerously short).

Kiwifruits are often bargain-priced in markets: choose those soft enough to yield to gentle pressure. Kiwifruit can be stored in the refrigerator and should be peeled

just before eating. Or you can eat them like a boiled egg – just cut off the tops and scoop out the pale green flesh with its small black seeds.

**Leeks** belong to the same family as garlic and onions, and share many of their qualities. But leeks have a pleasant blandness that is all their own. Their mild but distinctive flavour lends itself particularly well to warming, winter soups, where they combine happily with potatoes, onions, and carrots. Leek pies – in which stewed leeks and cream formed the filling – were popular in farmhouse cookery, as a side dish, to serve with the roast. Our Leek Pasties (see p.148) are a tasty hot or cold snack. When leeks are cheap and plentiful, pick the tender small ones, and use them for a salad. Clean the leeks and poach them in a mixture of oil, water, and aromatic herbs, then lift them out and leave to cool in the remainder of this liquid.

When you clean leeks, don't discard the green tops. Save the sounder leaves and make a vegetable stock with them.

**Lemons** People who recall the acute food shortages of World War II often single out lemons as the greatest deprivation. Lemons have a thousand uses in the preparation and presentation of food: in salad dressings, to enhance the flavour of other fruit (as in apple purées), or with avocados, to add a sharp note to

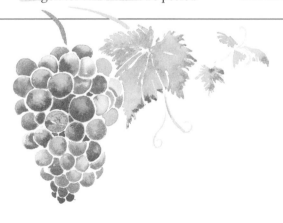

a bouquet of blander flavours, and in marinades for meat and fish. Their powerful antiseptic properties have probably saved many an oblivious diner from discomfort due to doubtful fish or oysters, and when the barman snaps a piece of lemon peel in two before dropping it in your cocktail, he's adding a drop of its essential oil to give extra pezazz. (You can see the oil floating in a tiny patch on the surface if you look.)

Lemons earned their reputation as a cure for scurvy (vitamin C deficiency) long before vitamin C itself was identified. They have plenty of vitamin C – twice as much as oranges – as well as bioflavonoids and B vitamins.

The lemon is thought of as a highly acid fruit, and for this reason is often forbidden to sufferers from rheumatism. In fact, its acidity is due to organic acids that are metabolized during digestion to produce potassium carbonate – which helps to neutralize excess acidity. Lemon juice is actually protective of the mucous membrane lining the digestive tract.

**Lentils,** like all dried legumes, are rich in useful minerals and trace elements, as well as vital B-complex vitamins. However, since they contain 23.8 per cent protein and 50.8 per cent starch, they are less easily digested than other foods, and should be eaten only occasionally on the Superfoods Diet, where they are treated, for this reason, as a neutral food. The combination of meat and legumes is particularly tough on the digestion. Most legumes combine more happily with starch foods than with protein foods and acid fruit.

**Lettuce,** in one form or another, is available all the year round, in ever-increasing variety, from the soft butterheads, through exotic oakleaf and red treviso varieties, to the crisp cos and the crunchy iceberg. But whatever kind of lettuce you eat, it must have one pre-eminent quality – freshness. A tired and wilted lettuce is a sorry object indeed. Ideally, a lettuce should be eaten the same day it is picked.

For suggestions on the perfect tossed green salad, turn to the Salads section on p.120–32. Lettuce supplies vitamins C and A – in the form of beta-carotene: the greener the better. In traditional medicine, lettuce is a cure for insomnia, whether eaten raw or braised. So don't serve Peas with Lettuce (see p.113) for a dinner party if your want the evening to be long and lively!

**Melons** are a cooling, delicious treat in hot weather: a large slice of crunchy pink watermelon – sold from roadside stands all over the Mediterranean – beats any canned fizzy drink for refreshment. A two-day monofast on melons of any kind is a delightful summer clean-out of the whole system.

Like grapes, melons of all kinds should be eaten on their own, or at least at the start of a meal, since they ferment rapidly in the stomach. Eating melon as a pudding, at the end of a substantial meal, is asking for digestive trouble.

**Millet** is rich in silicon, a structural part of collagen, the tough substance that holds us together. Silicon is vital for the health of hair, skin, teeth, eyes, and nails. Deficiency in this mineral can result in a sagging of connective tissue.

The only grain that is alkaline, millet is particularly suitable for invalids or growing children, and is easy on the digestion. A simple millet pilaff makes a pleasant change from rice or potatoes as the centrepiece of a starch meal, and lends itself well to spicy flavouring. Cold, it can be made into croquettes with the addition of egg yolk, onion, and herbs.

**Oats** have been the staple diet of some of the hardiest races – including the big-boned, well-developed, and mentally alert Scottish highlanders, and the inhabitants of the Hebrides. What makes oats such a splendid food?

Oats are richly nutritious, containing over 12 per cent protein by volume. They also contain polyunsaturated fats, a little vitamin E, and plenty of the B-complex vitamins. Oats are also spectacularly high in calcium, potassium, and magnesium – minerals that, like the B-complex vitamins, are vital to a healthy nervous system, as well as strong bones and teeth; and they supply plenty of silicon for healthy arterial walls. Recent research has shown, too, that oats help lower excess cholesterol levels. So eat porridge for breakfast – and you are doing your arteries a real favour.

The Scots themselves have firm ideas on how porridge should be made: with oatmeal, for a start, rather than with flakes. The oatmeal is added to briskly boiling water, stirred, then taken off the heat, and left to cook for 20 minutes or so. A little salt is added after 10 minutes, and pinches of fresh oatmeal are stirred in from time to time until it is done. Each breakfaster has his own bowl of cream – into which every spoonful of porridge is dipped. Oatcakes are another excellent way

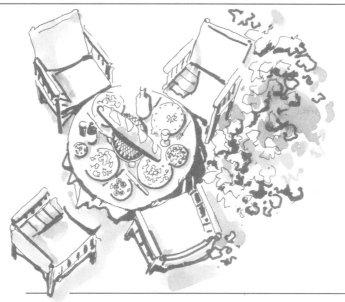

**Entertain your friends with a healthy and delicious feast of Superfoods**

to enjoy oats: eat them fresh and homemade, with thick winter soups, or put them in your packed lunch.

**Oily fish** Once high on the list of dieters' no-nos, oily fish like mackerel, salmon, herring, and anchovy are now known to contain high levels of eicosapentanoeic acid, one of a group of fatty acids belonging to the poetically named Omega-3 family, which are essential to healthy cell function, and thus vital to normal health. On the Superfoods Diet, you can disregard their high calorie count, and enjoy this delicious and ultra-healthy food.

**Olive oil** For years, nutritionists have been earnestly assuring us that the more highly polyunsaturated fats were, the better they were for our health. This put olive oil – a monounsaturated fat – way down the list. Research has now belatedly confirmed the peasant wisdom that all around the Mediterranean considered olive oil to be such a marvellous food-medicine.

Polyunsaturated fats can combine in the body with oxygen to form peroxides – otherwise known as free radicals. The more unsaturated the fat, the more free radicals may be created. These unstable compounds are highly destructive: they can seriously damage cell membranes, and even denature DNA. Without sufficient antioxidants – vitamins A,

C, and E among them – in the diet, polyunsaturated fats can actually be a threat to our health.

Olive oil is more easily digested than any other oil, and from 1992, EEC regulations will guarantee – as Italian law already does – that Extra Virgin Olive Oil has been mechanically extracted, and untreated by chemicals. This is more than you can say of any other oil, except for the pricey cold-pressed oils sold in health food shops.

Even disregarding its nutritional superiorities, it would be hard to resist making olive oil (if possible Extra Virgin) your choice for any dish where the flavour of the oil matters and is noticeable: pasta sauces, salad dressings, properly made mayonnaise, the scrumptious Italian snack *bruschetta*, and the Provençal *pan bagna* among them.

**Onions** Onions belong to the same botanical family as garlic. Like garlic, they have become the subject of intensive modern medical research, which only confirms the high reputation as a cure-all they have always enjoyed.

Eat plenty of onions in the winter – they'll keep you free of chesty colds. Children love onions baked in the oven like potatoes (test for doneness with a skewer pushed into the middle) and eaten with salt and butter. A purée of onions (see p.114) is a lovely accompaniment to a rich

meat or game dish, while on the other hand onions can add zest to blander foods, like rabbit or chicken: try our Chicken with Onions on p.102. When you have a cold or are hard hit by the winter blues, comfort yourself with creamy Onion and Garlic Soup (p.75).

**Oranges** Vitamin C, bioflavonoids, and beta-carotene are all present in an orange. Fresh and ripe, we'd eat it as if it were zero-rated, nutritionally, so delicious is it. Eat oranges whole rather than pressing their juice out and throwing the rest away. Oranges seem to have a natural affinity for other orange-coloured foods, for instance carrots. One of the most delicious dishes we have ever tasted is Salmon with Orange Sauce on p.91. Oranges make lovely salads, too: one of the great Mediterranean combinations is oranges with black olives and onions, served with a tangy lemon dressing. Oranges also go well with mint in salads – a more unexpected partnership.

**Pears** are a high-profile fruit on the Superfoods Diet since – as long as they are truly sweet and ripe – they can be eaten with Starch meals, thanks to their low acidity and high sugar content. Who, in any case, would want to eat any other kind of pear? Unripe pears can be turned into a pudding for a Protein meal by stewing in red wine with warm spices.

**Peas** are an immensely popular vegetable. We get through millions of cans and freezer packs annually. Fresh young peas, eaten as soon as possible after being picked, and lovingly hand-shelled, are another matter altogether. Once you have eaten and enjoyed them, you can understand how it was that when they were first introduced to Britain in the seventeenth century, they were considered as much a luxury as caviar is today. Peas supply useful amounts of B vitamins – more when they are fresh than when frozen or canned – as well as vitamins A and C.

**Peppers, sweet,** come rainbow-coloured these days – red, yellow, orange, green, and near-black. Their colour gives them wonderful eye-appeal, as well as indicating high levels of beta-carotene and vitamin C. Enjoy them in salads, either fresh or grilled and cooled, or bake them into a wonderful casserole (see p.108).

**Potatoes** must provide a pretty good nutritional package, since the Irish peasantry lived on almost nothing else for generations, without any obvious health problems. Boiled or baked this superfood supplies fibre, B complex, useful minerals, and just enough vitamin C to keep scurvy at bay, even during winter. Potatoes are one of the most appetizing and versatile of all vegetables. On the Superfoods Diet, they come into their own; no longer a mere adjunct to the roast or the stew, but the star of delicious dishes like the Potato Galette (see p.118). Potatoes can be a meal in themselves, needing little more than a green vegetable and a side salad to accompany them. A baked potato is hardly Fast Food, but it's certainly one of the simplest and most satisfying dishes we know.

**Pumpkin seeds** belong with Protein foods, because of their high protein content: they're also rich in zinc, iron, calcium, and some B vitamins. Around the Mediterranean, children shell and eat pumpkin seeds as happily as they do peanuts: we would do well to copy them.

**Rabbit** has gone up-market in recent years, and about time, too. Rabbit is much lower in fat than beef or lamb, and a smaller proportion of that fat is saturated. Quite apart from its low fat content, rabbit is seldom farmed in the dire conditions endured by poultry, and makes a delicious change from meat and poultry from time to time.

**Radishes** belong to the crucifer family. They are valued in traditional medicine as a tonic for the liver and gall bladder but once they become old, woody, and windy, they may turn into an irritant rather than a stimulant. To be enjoyed at their best, radishes should be picked and eaten straight out of the garden. The state of their leaves is a useful clue to their freshness: when these are still fresh and green, enjoy radishes, leaves and all. If the leaves are already wilted, don't bother. Radishes are nice eaten Middle Eastern-style as an appetizer. Serve little saucers of radishes, black olives, and little strips of celery, with wholewheat *pitas* or crusty rolls and butter.

**Raspberries** This tart, delectable fruit supplies not only a fair amount of vitamin C, but also useful amounts of calcium, potassium, iron, and magnesium – all vital to the convalescent, as well as to those suffering from heart problems, fatigue, or depression. All are easily absorbed thanks to that vitamin C.

Naturally astringent, raspberries can do you good along the whole length of your digestive tract, helping counter spongy, diseased gums, upset stomachs, and diarrhoea along the way.

Raspberries are another fruit best eaten on its own, or combined with other soft fruit such as blackcurrants, tiny *fraises de bois,* and strawberries.

**Rice** is a marvellous complete food, the dietary staple of the East, and until rice-milling arrived on the scene, it was eaten unpolished by all but the rich. Who eats brown rice in Eastern countries today? And the great risottos of Italy, like the paellas of Spain and the pilaus of the Middle East, are all based on white rice: many of them just aren't as good when made with the far healthier brown variety.

The compromise answer is "parboiled" or "converted" rice, which looks and behaves almost exactly like white rice, but has been subjected to a process of steaming that drives some of the vitamins back into the starchy grain.

Instead of trying to adapt recipes devised for white rice to the more solid and slow-cooking brown rice, however, it's better to enjoy this healthier foodstuff in dishes where its own qualities are respected – there are several among our recipes.

The most versatile of foodstuffs, rice needs little more than some oil or butter, herbs or spices, and perhaps a touch of onion, to make a wholesome and appetizing dish. You can build vegetable curries around it, or add it to soups; cooked and cold, you can make it into salads, or stuff vegetables with it. Add egg yolk, onions, and herbs to make little croquettes.

Here is a simple, foolproof way to cook brown rice. Wash it, then put it in a heavy casserole with a tight-fitting lid. Pour in enough boiling water to cover it with extra water to the depth of a thumbnail, and put it in a moderate oven for about 45 minutes. If it's still damp at this stage, remove the lid, turn the oven off, and let it dry out a little in the still warm oven. A friend of ours then puts it to bed until his guests are ready, wrapping the casserole in layers of rug or continental quilt to keep warm.

Plain, boiled brown rice, incidentally, is a universal folk remedy for diarrhoea. The water in which rice is boiled is also recommended for fevers. Rice has a beneficial soothing and cleansing effect on the entire intestinal tract.

Rice should be well washed in running water before cooking, but it should NEVER be soaked – whatever the recipe says – since vital minerals and vitamins leach out together with the dirt.

**Spinach** is rich in caretenoids – the plant precursors of vitamin A. Cancer research is increasingly focusing on the whole spectrum of carotenoids – not just beta-carotene – in dark green, or brightly coloured fruit and vegetables, and spinach is more highly endowed with these potential cancer-fighters even than carrots: a true Superfood.

Fresh spinach should be young, tender, and bright in colour. Wash it thoroughly, in several changes of water, to get rid of the last traces of grit. Then pack all the spinach into a big pan, cover tightly, and cook over the lowest flame, until the leaves have all wilted and begun to cook. Once cooked, strain, pressing

out every last drop of moisture. Chop roughly, adding a little butter and nutmeg, or olive oil and lemon juice.

**Sprouted seeds** are a wonderful source of vitamins and minerals: they have been described as "the most live, pure, nutritious food imaginable". They're also cheap, easy to grow – even if you don't own so much as a window-box – and always organically grown, without a trace of fertilizer or pesticide. Use sprouts to give a crunch to salads, and interest to sandwiches.

**Strawberries** are so delicious it's hard to believe how good they are for us, too. Their high iron content makes them therapeutic for anaemia and fatigue. People with skin problems should enjoy plenty of this wonderful fruit, which cleanses and regenerates the intestinal flora.

Like grapes, melons, and other soft fruit, strawberries ferment rapidly in the stomach. They are best eaten at the start of a meal, or better still, on their own: a wonderful breakfast.

Perhaps no other fruit shows up more clearly the advantages of eating fruit and vegetables that have been sunripened and locally grown. What can compare with the wonderful flavour of strawberries locally grown on a hot summer's

day? Certainly not strawberries that have journeyed great distances from Spain, Italy, or Israel.

**Tomatoes** Strictly speaking, tomatoes are fruit rather than vegetable. They count as neutral for the Superfoods Diet, unless they are cooked, when chemical changes increase their acidity, and make them unsuitable for consumption with starch dishes. Fresh, deep-red, sunripened tomatoes are one of the treats of summer. Enjoy them raw in salads, or in deliciously fresh uncooked sauces for pasta or rice (see p.94).

**Turkey** Once an annual Christmas treat, turkey is now available all the year round, and grows in popularity all the time. It's cheaper than veal, although the turkey breast and escalopes can replace veal in a number of popular recipes: Turkey Tonnato, for instance. It's also very low in fat – roast turkey contains a mere 1 per cent saturated fat.

**Turnips** are an underrated vegetable, one of the lesser known members of the great crucifer family. They were certainly prized in traditional medicine: a thin purée of turnips, cooked in milk, is an old country remedy for bronchitis. A rather creamier purée is a delicious accompaniment to game, or rabbit;

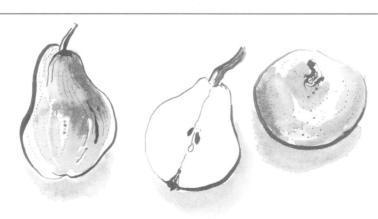

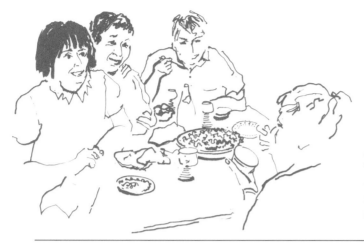

**All the family will enjoy the Superfoods Diet**

and the distinctive earthy taste of turnips would be sadly missed from the classic *navarin printanier* – that wonderful French lamb stew enriched with all the new baby vegetables of springtime. Turnips make a lovely soup, too (see Turnip Soup with Dill, p.80).

**Walnuts,** the most nutritious of all the nuts, contain more than 10 per cent protein by weight. They also supply zinc, iron, magnesium, potassium, B vitamins, and some vitamin E. They are rich in polyunsaturated fats, and should therefore be eaten with foods that contain antioxidants, like fruit and salads. Eat them fresh from the shell when in season – towards the end of the year – when their sweet, nutty flavour is at its finest. Don't touch walnuts if they taste rancid.

**Watercress** is another richly nutritious member of the potent crucifer family, other members of which are cabbages, broccoli, brussels sprouts, radishes, turnip, horseradish, and kale. Like them, watercress is rich in both vitamin A and vitamin C. In the depths of winter, its crisp tang is welcome in salads, or in velvety soups. Throughout the year, watercress is a useful salad ingredient, teaming successfully with oranges, apples, chicory, and avocados.

**Wheat** If millions of people made no other change in their diet than to switch from white to wholemeal bread, they would still be staggered by the improvement in their health and general vitality. Farmers and millers profit handsomely from milling the goodness out of nutrient-rich wholewheat: they can sell the wheatgerm and the once despised bran to health food shops.

Although a quarter of lost nutrients milled out of white flour is replaced, there are other important losses that are not made good – of nutrients which may well be in short supply in the modern diet, such as zinc, magnesium, vitamin $B_6$, or the vital antioxidant vitamin E. Wholewheat and the bread made from it is a Superfood. Refined wheat – like white rice – is not.

By all means enjoy a wonderful French *baguette* – or a plate of pasta made from white flour – as an occasional treat; just make sure that the rest of your diet is well supplied with Superfoods.

**Wheatgerm** should be absolutely fresh, preferably vacuum-packed: once opened, refrigerate it and eat up quickly. Because of its high content of vitamin E-rich oil, it can turn rancid very quickly, when it becomes an actively perilous food. Taste it: if it's not fresh and nutty, return it to the suppliers.

Wheatgerm is a rich source of vitamin E and the B vitamins; however, as a concentrated foodstuff it should not be eaten to excess. On the Superfoods Diet wheatgerm is neutral, and can replace breadcrumbs in protein-based croquettes or burgers.

**Yogurt** How can something so delicious be so good for you? Yogurt doesn't just taste nice – the rich, creamy Greek-style ones, especially – it does a wonderful spring-cleaning job down in your gut, where it helps keep the balance between friendly and unfriendly bacteria tipped firmly in your favour. If you've been taking antibiotics, yogurt should be written into the prescription, too.

The lactic acids in yogurt act on the digestion in several ways. They synthesize some of the B vitamins, biotin, folic acid, and $B_{12}$. They increase the uptake of calcium and magnesium, and their presence in the intestines checks the proliferation of pathogenic bacteria. Even people who can't digest milk – an estimated 40 per cent of the Western population – can normally cope with yogurt.

Plain yogurt is an excellent substitute for cream: all that smooth richness but far fewer calories. It can be stirred into cold summer soups to give a coolly creamy effect. Yogurt is also an ingredient in light, tart dressings for salads.

## HERBS & SPICES

The herbs and spices used in traditional cookery around the world play a vital role in the Superfoods Diet. They add savour, piquancy, zest, and interest to dozens of dishes, and almost all have a beneficial effect on the digestion. A digestion that functions sweetly and efficiently is the cornerstone of the Superfoods Diet.

**Basil** is the traditional accompaniment to tomatoes in Mediterranean cookery, and an ingredient of the lovely green Italian pasta sauce *pesto – pistou* in Provence. Basil is an expensive item in supermarkets, but many greengrocers sell whole plants. Carefully tended with lots of watering, and all the sun available, a good plant should see you right through the fresh tomato season.

**Bay** The distinctive flavour of bay leaves is an intrinsic part of the classic French *bouquet garni*. Bay leaves are prized for their antiseptic properties and for their assistance to the digestion.

**Caraway** In Central Europe, caraway seeds are a well-known aid to digestion: people chew a few of them before sitting down to a rich meal. Like dill, which contains the same compound, *carvone,* they are particularly effective for coping with wind or flatulence. In North European cookery they are often added to dishes containing cabbage, chick peas, or beans.

**Chilli peppers** are used whole, either fresh or dried, or in the form of dried flakes, or dried and powdered, or in the popular formulation known as cayenne pepper. Chillies are popular the world over, in Central and South America, China, the Middle East, and wherever people like their food with a real kick to it.

In Italy every street market sells bundles of the little fiery red peppers to hang up in your kitchen, for use in dozens of dishes, including pasta. Try hot chilli flavours in Fish with a Fiery Sauce (see p.90), Red Hot Chicken (see p.100), or Piquant Red Sauce for pasta (see p.140). Go easy at first, until you know just how much you can take. The fiery little peppers should be prepared under running water, when fresh; just a whiff of their volatile oil can make your nose and throat burn. Slit the pods open, remove ALL the seeds, dry in a paper towel, and use with caution! (Rinse your hands carefully afterwards.) The dried ones are less lethal and can be used whole – although they are usually fished out once they have made their emphatic contribution to the dish being cooked. Try a flake or two of chilli in soups, in dried bean dishes, in tomato sauces, and with vegetables such as cauliflower, potatoes, and green beans.

**Chives** are members of the onion family, and have the same zest to their flavour, although in a mild form. Use them lavishly in the summer, snipped into salads, or as a garnish for cold soups.

**Cinnamon** lends its delicate but distinct flavour to dozens of minced meat or chicken dishes in Middle Eastern cookery. It has a strong antiseptic action, which is useful in hot countries where refrigerators are far from commonplace. It's one of the warming spices particularly useful in winter: lovely with cooked apples, or any kind of stewed fruit. Add a sprinkling to plain yogurt with honey and nuts, too.

**Cloves**, like cinnamon, are warming and antiseptic. Everyone uses cloves with apples – but try adding one to a beef stew for a change.

**Coriander** seeds are an essential ingredient of curry powders, and for those cold appetizers cooked *à la grecque*. Powdered, they add a distinctive North African flavour to meat and fish dishes. In hot, stimulating food, this mild spice is valued for its cooling quality, and its assistance to the digeston. Fresh, green coriander was introduced into Britain by the Romans, and widely used up to Elizabethan times, when its popularity waned. Now it is once more available, thanks to the huge demand from West Indian and Pakistani communities: experiment with it in fish and vegetable dishes.

**Cumin seeds** Another curry herb, but the incomparable smell given off by the warmed, crushed seeds evokes Middle Eastern cookery, too. Use it in rich, fried dishes or with beans to counter flatulence and dyspepsia.

**Dill** This pretty, feathery herb is a favourite accompaniment to fish in Scandinavian cookery. Dried, it is a piquant addition to bland cheeses like Mozzarella, or to salad dressings. Babies taste dill in the form of gripe water, where it is highly effective. Its name actually comes from a Saxon word meaning "to lull": an apt name for a herb so soothing to the digestive tract.

**Fennel** The dark green fronds of this herb are a classic ingredient of the *court-bouillon* of fish dishes and soups. Add fresh fronds of fennel to the mayonnaise you serve with cold fish in summer. Fennel goes particularly well with rich fish like mackerel, and a great French gastronomic treat is sea bass grilled on a bed of dried fennel branches, served with a buttery sauce. Use the feathery fronds sprouting from fennel bulbs as a garnish for salads. Fennel is an excellent aid to a troubled digestion.

**Ginger** This warming, antiseptic herb is widely used in the cookery of meat and fish in the Far East, where it helps counter putrefaction. It's almost as popular as a sweet spice in the West. Use the fresh root whenever possible: dried ginger is poor stuff by comparison. Like the other warming spices, ginger aids the digestion.

**Horseradish** Traditionally made up in jars and eaten with roast beef, horseradish deserves to be more adventurously used. Try the fresh root grated into salad dressing, mayonnaise, or cottage cheese, or add a little to natural yogurt as an accompaniment to smoked fish. Horseradish is an invigorating herb: powerfully stimulating to the digestion – a good reason for eating it with rich foods like roast beef.

**Marjoram** Sweet or pot marjoram is the gentler garden variety of wild marjoram or oregano (see below), and has similar qualities. Fresh, it has a lovely sweet aroma, which comes over well in omelettes: experiment with it, too, in soups, and in salad dressings.

**Mint** There are many varieties of mint, a popular herb for flavouring light summer dishes, and justly famous for its wonderfully calming effect on the digestive tract. Mint deserves to be more widely used than in the clichéd mint sauce (itself often a horrid vinegary concoction). Add it very finely chopped, and plentifully, to a tossed green salad.

Mint is a natural partner to fresh tomato and cucumber; and, therefore, an important ingredient of the delicious Middle Eastern cracked wheat salad, *Tabbouleh*.

**Nutmeg,** familiar from so many favourite winter sweet treats, can have a mildly uplifting effect in small doses and it is also good for the digestion. Don't overdo it as, in large quantities, it can have an hallucinogenic effect.

**Oregano** is the distinctive note in that wonderful pizza smell – an obliging herb that is almost as delicious dried as it is fresh. Like many other aromatic herbs, it is an effective antiseptic for the respiratory tract, so enjoy plenty of oregano in winter.

**Parsley** is rich in vitamins A and C, and in iron, calcium, and potassium, as well as lifegiving chlorophyll. Use parsley fresh and use it lavishly.

Herbalists value parsley for its diuretic action: parsley tea was used in the trenches of World War I for soldiers suffering kidney complications following dysentery. Parsley helps eliminate uric acid, making it useful in rheumatism and gout. Parsley tea was an old country aid to digestion: Maurice Messegué recalls the monster pot brewed by his grandmother, Sophie, after a Lucullan feast of *foie gras*, roast chicken, sautéed mushrooms, crêpes, custards, and apple tart. Add a bunch of fresh parsley whenever you make a freshly pressed vegetable juice.

**Rosemary,** that inseparable companion of roast lamb and chicken in Mediterranean cookery, is a powerful friend to the digestive system, prompting production of extra bile for fat digestion.

**Sage** and onion stuffing for roast goose is true kitchen medicine. Sage aids the digestion of rich, heavy food. Italian cooks always add a leaf of sage to the pan when they fry sausages or pork.

**Savory, summer** The German name of this peppery little plant means "bean herb", since it eases the digestion of beans, split peas, broad beans, and lentils, as well as benefiting the entire digestive tract. It has an antiseptic action on the gut.

**Tarragon** The delicate, distinctive flavour of this herb seems peculiarly French; used with roast chicken, in sauces, in omelettes, to flavour a wine vinegar. The dried herb is a pale shadow of the fresh. Another of the culinary herbs which aids the digestion, tarragon can help relieve gas, flatulence, and acidity.

**Thyme** contributes the deepest aromatic note in a *bouquet garni*, and it would be hard to imagine a robust peasant *daube* of beef, or a spring lamb stew without this wonderful herb. Thyme is also a powerful antiseptic and a general stimulant to the body's natural resistance, with marked anti-viral and anti-bacterial activity. Enjoy its distinctive flavour in food for cold, grey winter days, when your resistance is low.

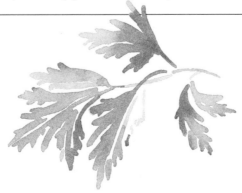

# THE RECIPES

All the recipes are for four people, unless otherwise stated.
The symbol beside each recipe indicates whether the content
of the dish is primarily protein or starch. Neutral dishes can
accompany protein or starch meals.

Recipe titles followed by a ★ are not suitable if you're
following the Intensive Weight Loss plan.

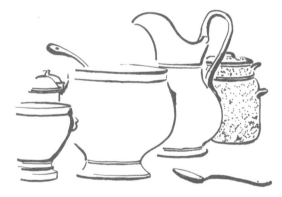

## STARTERS FOR PROTEIN MEALS

### NECTARINE AND PINK GRAPEFRUIT ON LETTUCE WITH SOUR CREAM DRESSING

PROTEIN

Wash and dry the nectarines, halve, remove the stones, and cut into thick slices. Peel the grapefruit, and split into segments, removing most of the thick white pith. Clean and shred the lettuce, and make a bed of it on a pretty serving dish. Arrange the nectarine slices and grapefruit segments alternately on top, cover with a damp cloth, and chill. Stir the pineapple juice and honey into the soured cream. Whisk it well, and just before serving, drizzle it over the fruit.

| INGREDIENTS |
| --- |
| 2 firm, ripe nectarines |
| 1 large pink grapefruit |
| lettuce leaves |
| 4tbs sour cream |
| 2tbs pineapple juice |
| 1tsp clear honey |

### AUBERGINE CAVIAR

PROTEIN

Heat the oven to 200°C/400°F/gas 6. Bake the aubergines until they are soft. Cut them open, scrape the flesh out into a bowl, add the lemon juice, and beat in the oil, drop by drop, until you have a fine, smooth cream. Crush the garlic and stir it in. Stir in the yogurt. Season to taste with freshly ground pepper and sea salt. Crush the coriander seeds and add. Stir once more, then cover the bowl, and chill for at least an hour.

| INGREDIENTS |
| --- |
| 2 large aubergines |
| juice of 1 large lemon |
| 3tbs extra-virgin olive oil |
| 1 fat clove garlic |
| 2tbs plain yogurt |
| salt and pepper |
| 5–6 coriander seeds |

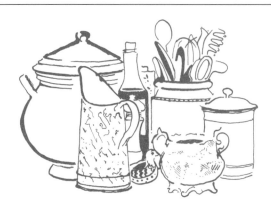

## MARINATED KIPPER FILLETS

### INGREDIENTS

| |
|---|
| 8–10 boneless kipper fillets (avoid the highly coloured ones) |
| 1tsp peppercorns |
| 1 bay leaf |
| juice of 1 large lemon |
| 1 small onion |
| 2tbs extra-virgin olive oil |

Prepare this dish in the morning for the evening, or leave overnight. Arrange the fillets on a long white china dish. Sprinkle over them the peppercorns and the bay leaf, torn into several pieces. Pour over the lemon juice. Leave to marinate. Just before serving, slice the onion, arrange several rings on top, and pour over the olive oil.

PROTEIN

## AUBERGINE AND TOMATO SALAD★

### INGREDIENTS

| |
|---|
| 2 medium aubergines |
| sea salt |
| 8 firm, ripe tomatoes – about 500g/1lb in all |
| extra-virgin olive oil |
| 1 glass dry white wine |
| 2 cloves garlic, crushed |
| 1tbs chopped fresh basil |

*The recipe for this unusual and delicious dish comes from one of our favourite cookery books:* Leaves From Our Tuscan Kitchen *by Janet Ross and Michael Waterfield.*

Peel the aubergines, remove the stalks, slice fairly thickly, and leave in a colander, sprinkled generously with sea salt, for the bitter juices to drain off. Peel the tomatoes – dip them in boiling water for a minute or two until the skins slide off easily – then slice. Arrange them on a serving dish.

PROTEIN

Heat the oil in a frying-pan, and fry the aubergine slices, turning them quickly – they should be tender but not browned. Remove from the pan as they are done. When they are all ready, put them back in the pan, pour over the white wine, and add the garlic and the basil. Let the liquid bubble and reduce, then pour the contents of the pan over the tomatoes. Leave to cool – but it should not be ice-cold. Just before serving, decorate with a little fresh basil.

## SALADE NIÇOISE

PROTEIN

*You can add cooked green beans, spring onions, and radishes to this dish, or to make it a more substantial meal, add chunks of tuna. If you want to serve it with a Starch meal, perhaps as a light luncheon, omit the anchovies, and use only the yolks of the eggs. Boiled new potatoes are another possible extra.*

Wash the lettuce, dry, and arrange in a salad bowl. Arrange attractively on top the eggs, peeled and quartered; the tomatoes, washed and quartered; the pepper, washed, cleaned of its seeds and flesh ribs, and sliced; the cucumber, peeled and cut into chunks; the anchovies, cut into smaller pieces, and the black olives. At this point, put a damp cloth over the bowl and place in a cool place until you are ready to serve the dish.

Make a dressing with the finely chopped garlic, oil, vinegar, and seasoning. Pour it over the salad at the last minute.

| INGREDIENTS |
| --- |
| 1 head of crisp lettuce |
| 2 hard-boiled eggs |
| 4 firm red tomatoes |
| 1 large red pepper |
| ½ cucumber |
| 4 anchovy fillets (soaked in milk for half an hour to remove excess saltiness) |
| 12 black olives |
| 2 cloves garlic |
| 3tbs extra-virgin olive oil |
| 1tbs tarragon wine vinegar |
| a pinch of *herbes de provence* |
| salt and pepper |

## WATERCRESS SOUP

PROTEIN

*The addition of yogurt makes this a soup to be eaten with a protein meal. Substitute a tablespoon – or less – of single cream, and you can enjoy it with a starch meal. This is a very light, fragrant green broth, cooked only for minutes in order to preserve the fresh taste of watercress and herbs. It needs no seasoning.*

Wash and trim the watercress, and add it to the stock, together with the parsley and mint. Cook gently for a few minutes, then put in a food processor or blender, and blend briefly. Reheat, beat in the yogurt with a wooden spoon, and serve hot.

Watercress soup can also be served cold – in which case beat in the yogurt just before you serve it.

| INGREDIENTS |
| --- |
| 2 bunches of watercress |
| 900ml/1½pts light vegetable stock |
| 1 tbs fresh chopped parsley |
| 1 tbs fresh mint leaves |
| 2tbs creamy yogurt |

# GAZPACHO

## INGREDIENTS

| |
| --- |
| 500g/1lb ripe tomatoes (they must be fresh) |
| 1 medium cucumber |
| 1 small onion |
| 1 green pepper |
| 1 clove garlic |
| 1 lemon |
| ½tsp white wine vinegar |
| 1tsp olive oil |
| salt and freshly ground pepper |
| ice cubes |

PROTEIN

*This particularly refreshing version of the famous Spanish soup is ideal for summer lunches.*

Peel the tomatoes (if you cover them in boiling water for a couple of minutes the skins will slide off easily). Save one, put the rest in a food processor, and whizz. Wash the cucumber, cut off a chunk, then peel and deseed. Clean and slice the onion, the green pepper, and the garlic – but save a chunk of the pepper, too – add them all to the food processor, and blend. Pour into a bowl, add the vinegar, season to taste, cover, and put in the refrigerator. Scrub the lemon, remove a long, paper-thin curl of its rind, then squeeze out the juice. Cut the reserved tomato, cucumber, green pepper, and lemon rind into very small dice. Put into a small bowl, moisten with the lemon juice and olive oil, and place in the refrigerator. Chill both for 4–5 hours.

Just before serving, combine the mixtures. Serve in glass bowls with a couple of ice cubes.

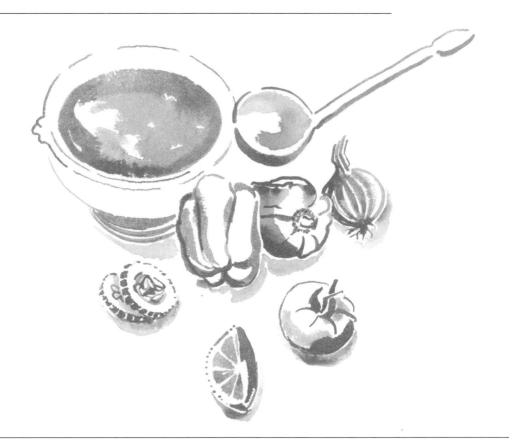

# APPLE AND WATERCRESS SOUP

**PROTEIN**

Peel, core, and slice the apples. Heat the stock, add the apples, and simmer until they are soft. Meanwhile, wash the watercress and trim off the stalks. Reserve enough leaves for use as a garnish, and add the rest to the apple stock. Simmer for a few minutes more, then purée in a blender or food processor. Add the lemon juice, season to taste, and leave to chill.

To serve, pour into 4 bowls, add a swirl of yogurt to each, and scatter the watercress leaves on top.

### INGREDIENTS

**6 eating apples (slightly tart varieties are better than the softer, blander apples)**

**1.2litres/2pts light chicken or vegetable stock**

**2 bunches watercress**

**juice of 1 lemon**

**salt and pepper**

**4tbs creamy yogurt**

# BEETROOT AND APPLE SOUP

**PROTEIN**

*This recipe can be made with cooked beetroot, to produce a pleasant summer soup. However, the tart earthiness of raw beetroot tastes even better and creates a brilliant red soup.*

Peel and grate the raw beetroot. Peel and finely chop the onion. Put both in a blender or food processor with a cupful of the apple juice, purée until smooth, and stir in the rest of the juice. Season to taste with salt and pepper, and chill. Serve in individual bowls – glass ones, if possible, for this good-looking dish. Swirl in the cream.

### INGREDIENTS

**500g/1lb uncooked beetroot**

**1 onion**

**600ml/1pt unsweetened apple juice**

**1tsp lemon juice**

**salt and freshly ground black pepper**

**150ml/¼pt sour or single cream**

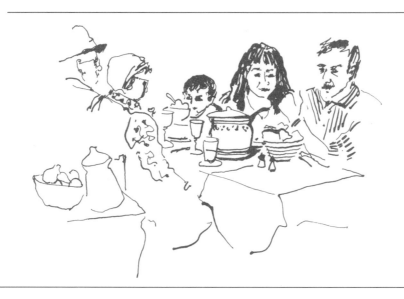

# CARROT, GINGER, AND ORANGE SOUP★

### INGREDIENTS

**450ml/¾pt light chicken or vegetable stock**

**375g/12oz young carrots, scraped and finely chopped**

**a little freshly grated ginger**

**150ml/¼pt freshly pressed orange juice**

**grated rind of 1 orange, carefully scrubbed**

**150ml/¼pt Greek yogurt**

**salt and pepper**

**2tsp coarsely grated orange rind**

Put the stock and carrots in a pan, bring to the boil, and simmer until the carrots are tender. Cool, then put in a blender or food processor with the grated ginger, orange juice, yogurt, and seasoning. Chill for at least 5 hours. Put in a pretty bowl or 4 soup cups. Serve decorated with the grated orange rind.

PROTEIN

# TART APPLE SLAW

### INGREDIENTS

**½ small white cabbage**

**150g/5oz plain yogurt**

**2tbs cream**

**1tsp grated horseradish**

**2 crisp eating apples**

**juice of 1 lemon**

**salt and pepper**

Clean the cabbage, shred very finely, wash, drain, and blot dry. Put the yogurt in a small bowl. Stir in the cream, and the grated horseradish. Peel the apples, and grate them into another bowl. Add the lemon juice, mix, and stir into the yogurt. Arrange the shredded cabbage on an attractive dish – a green one is especially nice – and spoon this sharp, creamy sauce over it.

PROTEIN

## STILTON EGGS★

**PROTEIN**

Cut the eggs in half lengthways. Remove the yolks and mash with the remaining ingredients. Pile the filling back into the egg whites, and top each half with a strip of anchovy. Serve on lettuce leaves.

| INGREDIENTS |
| --- |
| 4 hard-boiled eggs |
| 2tbs double cream |
| 50g/2oz stilton – a good moist one – or gorgonzola cheese |
| a pinch of salt |
| a pinch of chilli pepper |
| To garnish: |
| 8 anchovy strips |
| lettuce leaves |

## COURGETTE, GARLIC, AND BLUE CHEESE SOUP★

**PROTEIN**

*For a strong blue cheese flavour, choose stilton, gorgonzola, or danish blue. For a milder flavour, use blue brie or dolcelatte.*

Fry the onion and the garlic in a large pan with the butter until just soft. Add the courgettes and continue cooking, stirring frequently for about 10 minutes. Pour in the stock, add salt and pepper to taste, and the oregano, then bring to the boil. Lower the heat to a simmer, and continue cooking gently, stirring occasionally for about 20 minutes.

Remove any rind from the cheese, and chop it roughly. Process with the cream until smooth – save a little cream to swirl into the soup before serving. Add the soup to the food processor, and blend with the cheese and cream purée. (This may need to be done in 2 batches.)

Return the soup to a clean pan and reheat gently. Check and adjust the seasoning. Serve with an extra swirl of cream, sprinkled with the parsley.

| INGREDIENTS |
| --- |
| 1 medium onion, peeled and chopped |
| 2 cloves garlic, peeled and crushed |
| 35g/1½oz butter |
| 500g/1lb courgettes, washed, trimmed, and sliced |
| 1.2 litres/2pts homemade vegetable stock (or use a good vegetable stock cube) |
| salt and freshly ground black pepper |
| 2 sprigs of fresh oregano or a good pinch of dried |
| 125g/4oz blue cheese of your choice |
| 150ml/5fl oz single cream |
| chopped fresh parsley |

## PRAWNS WITH PINK GRAPEFRUIT

### INGREDIENTS

| |
|---|
| 250g/8oz peeled prawns (if frozen, defrost, and drain well) |
| 2 level tsp chopped fresh chives |
| 2 level tsp chopped fresh mint |
| 2tbs white wine vinegar |
| 1 large pink grapefruit |
| mixed green lettuce leaves (iceberg, frisée, etc) |
| To garnish: |
| lemon wedges |
| slices of cucumber |

Sprinkle the prawns with the chives, mint, and vinegar, and leave to marinate for about 45 minutes. Peel the grapefruit, remove all the pith and skin, and divide into segments. Wash and dry the lettuce, and put it on a serving dish. Arrange the segments on it, top with the prawns, and chill. Garnish with the lemon wedges and the cucumber.

**PROTEIN**

## ONION AND GARLIC SOUP

### INGREDIENTS

| |
|---|
| 4 medium onions or 2 large ones |
| 4 fat cloves garlic |
| 25g/1oz butter |
| 900ml/1½pts milk |
| 2 egg yolks |
| freshly ground black pepper |
| sea salt |
| nutmeg |

*This is a warm, comforting soup for a winter's day, which will also help keep coughs and colds at bay.*

Clean and slice the onions, and finely chop the garlic. Melt the butter in a heavy saucepan. Over a very gentle heat, sauté the onions and garlic until they are just beginning to colour: don't let them brown. Pour over the milk, and let it come very slowly to the boil. Purée or blend, and away from the heat, take a couple of spoonfuls of the soup and combine it with the well-beaten egg yolks. Return the soup to the pan, season with pepper and salt to taste, and reheat, taking care not to let it boil. Serve with a grating of nutmeg over the surface.

**PROTEIN**

# STARTERS FOR PROTEIN OR STARCH MEALS

## BORSCHT

**NEUTRAL**

*If you are serving Borscht as a starter to a Starch meal, omit the lemon juice, or greatly reduce it, and add a swirl of sour cream, not yogurt.*

Peel the beetroot and slice into thin strips. Heat the butter and oil in a heavy-bottomed pan, sweat the onion, then add the beetroot, carrots, celery, and fennel. Sauté over a very low heat for a few minutes, then add the stock and the herbs. Bring to the boil, turn down the heat, and simmer until the vegetables are soft – about 30 minutes.

Strain into another pan, purée the vegetables in a blender or food processor, and return them to the soup. Serve hot or chilled, with a swirl of yogurt or sour cream.

| INGREDIENTS |
| --- |
| 500g/1lb raw beetroot |
| 25g/1oz butter |
| 1tbs olive oil |
| 1 medium onion, sliced |
| 2 carrots, peeled and sliced |
| 2 stalks celery, chopped |
| 1.2 litres/2pt vegetable stock |
| thyme, parsley, and bay leaf |
| salt and pepper |
| juice of 1 lemon |
| 1–2tbs sour cream or plain yogurt |

## KEKI'S LEEK AND LENTIL SOUP

**NEUTRAL**

Boil the lentils in half the water until they are soft. Add the rest of the water and all the other ingredients, except for the vegetable bouillon powder, and simmer for 10–15 minutes. Blend. Add vegetable bouillon powder to taste and serve.

| INGREDIENTS |
| --- |
| 175g/6oz red lentils |
| 1litre/1¾pts water |
| 250g/8oz leeks, cleaned, trimmed, and finely sliced |
| 1 medium onion, finely chopped |
| 1 clove garlic, chopped |
| 1 small piece of green pepper, chopped |
| 1 sprig of parsley |
| 1–2tsp vegetable bouillon powder |

## BEANFEAST BROTH

### INGREDIENTS

| |
|---|
| **250g/8oz dried beans – pick your favourites** |
| **1 litre/1¾pts water** |
| **4 medium carrots, washed and sliced** |
| **1 turnip, peeled and chopped** |
| **2 celery stalks with some of the leaves, chopped** |
| **1 onion, finely chopped** |
| **4 or 5 mushrooms, cleaned and finely chopped** |
| **2tsp tomato purée** |
| **black pepper** |
| **fresh herbs – summer or winter savory, chervil, parsley, pot marjoram, finely chopped, and *bouquet garni*** |
| **a dash of *shoyu* or *tamari*** |
| **1tbs finely chopped fresh parsley, to garnish** |

**NEUTRAL**

Soak the beans overnight in some of the water. Put the beans and their soaking water, together with the rest of the water, in a big pan. Bring to the boil, and boil briskly for 10 minutes. Turn down the heat, and simmer steadily until the beans are done.

Drain off the cooking water into another pan. Add the vegetables, stir in the tomato purée, and add the freshly ground black pepper and the herbs. Bring to the boil, turn down the heat, and simmer until the vegetables are cooked. Return the beans to the pan. Check the seasoning – for a change, add a dash of *shoyu* or *tamari*. Heat through, and serve, garnished with the parsley.

## CHILLED FENNEL SOUP★

### INGREDIENTS

| |
|---|
| **2 heads of fennel** |
| **1tsp fennel seeds** |
| **900ml/1½pts chicken or light vegetable stock** |
| **salt and white pepper** |
| **2tbs double cream** |

**NEUTRAL**

Quarter the cleaned heads of fennel – reserve a few fronds to use as a decoration for the soup. Simmer the fennel, together with the fennel seeds, in the stock, until it is tender. Drain the fennel, reserving the cooking liquid, and blend or process to a thick purée, with a little of this liquid. Then add the rest of the liquid and leave to cool. Half an hour before serving, stir in the double cream, and chill again. Serve decorated with some of the pretty green fronds of fennel.

# ALMOND AND CARROT CREAM★

**NEUTRAL**

Trim and clean the carrots, onion, celery, and leek. Slice them all very finely. Heat the butter in a heavy pan, add the vegetables, and let them take on a little colour. Add half the almonds, and turn them over in the butter. Add the stock, and bring to the boil. Turn down the heat, and simmer for about half an hour.

Put the soup in a food processor or blender, and process to a smooth cream. Return to the pan, and bring back to the boil. Remove from the heat, add the cream, grate in a little nutmeg, and season to taste. Serve hot, with the remaining almonds scattered over the surface.

| INGREDIENTS |
| --- |
| 500g/1lb carrots |
| 1 spring onion |
| 1 celery stalk |
| 1 leek |
| 50g/2oz butter |
| 125g/4oz peeled almonds, coarsely ground |
| 1 litre/1¾pt light vegetable stock |
| 150ml/5fl oz single cream |
| grated nutmeg |
| salt and pepper |

# MEZE

**NEUTRAL**

As you sip your drink in a Greek taverna, or wait for dinner to arrive, you could be served a selection of little savoury appetizers and a basket of hot *pita* bread. *Meze* can include salads like the cucumber, mint, and yogurt *tsatsiki*, aubergine purées of different kinds, *taramasalata* – that creamy fish roe paste, *hummus* – the chickpea purée, and pieces of grilled cheese. The very simplest *meze*, however, can consist of just a selection of fresh vegetables. If it's a Starch meal, provide hot wholewheat *pita* bread with them. If it's Protein, Aubergine Caviar (p.68) is a pleasant addition to *meze*. You can also serve them with the simplest dip of all: a little extra-virgin olive oil, and sea salt. Choose from any of the suggested ingredients, whatever is in season.

| INGREDIENTS |
| --- |
| black olives |
| whole fresh radishes, with their green stalks on |
| spring onions |
| strips of baby carrot |
| small chunks of fennel |
| strips of celery |
| whole red cherry tomatoes |

# STARTERS FOR STARCH MEALS

## THICK VEGETABLE SOUP WITH BARLEY

### INGREDIENTS

| |
|---|
| 2tbs oil |
| 1 large onion, sliced |
| 2 cloves garlic, finely chopped |
| 2 large carrots, cleaned and thinly sliced |
| 2 medium potatoes, scrubbed and diced |
| 2tbs pot barley, well washed |
| salt and pepper |
| fresh chopped parsley, to garnish |

Heat the oil, then add the onion and garlic, and cook until translucent – don't let them turn brown. Add the carrots, potatoes, and barley. Stir them about in the oil, then pour in the stock and bring to the boil. Check the seasoning, and simmer for 30–40 minutes, until the vegetables and barley are cooked. Serve this soup sprinkled with plenty of chopped parsley.

STARCH

## JERUSALEM ARTICHOKE CREAM★

### INGREDIENTS

| |
|---|
| 500g/1lb Jerusalem artichokes |
| iced water, with a dash of lemon or vinegar |
| 1 large onion |
| 1tbs butter |
| 750ml/1¼pts light vegetable stock |
| 2–3tbs single cream |
| 1tbs very finely chopped parsley |
| freshly ground pepper |

Peel the artichokes, and put them into the acidulated water to stop them discolouring, until you are ready to use them. Finely chop the onion, melt the butter in a heavy pan, and fry the onion over a moderate heat until it is translucent – don't let it change colour. Drain and dry the artichokes, slice very finely, and add to the onions in the pan. Turn the heat right down, cover tightly, and leave to cook for 10–15 minutes until the artichokes are soft. Check from time to time that nothing is starting to burn. Purée in a blender or food processor with a little of the stock, return to the pan, and add the rest of the stock. Just before serving, stir in the cream. Sprinkle a little chopped parsley on top, and a shake of pepper.

STARCH

# TURNIP SOUP WITH DILL

**STARCH**

Prepare the turnips – which should be as fresh and young as possible. Have a pan of cold water ready with a dash of vinegar or lemon juice in it, to prevent the turnips from discolouring before you are ready to use them. Top and tail them, and peel them. Quarter them, and then halve the quarters and put these in the acidulated water.

Peel and finely chop the onion. Melt the butter in a thick pan, add the onions, and turn the heat down to very low. Cover the pan and leave the onions to sweat until they are translucent and just beginning to colour (shake the pan from time to time, and check that the onions are not sticking). Then add the turnips, drained and dried, a sprinkling of salt and freshly ground pepper, and the dill – reserve a little of the dill for garnishing the soup. Cover the pan tightly again and put back over a low heat to sweat for about half an hour – so that the vegetables cook gently in their own steam.

Add the stock, and let it heat through gently. Put the soup in a food processor or blender, and blend to a smooth texture. Reheat the soup gently, stir in the cream, and serve with a couple of feathery dill leaves arranged on top.

| INGREDIENTS |
| --- |
| 500g/1lb young turnips |
| 1 medium onion |
| 1tbs butter |
| salt and pepper |
| a bunch of fresh dill |
| 900ml/1½pts light vegetable stock or water |
| 1tbs cream |

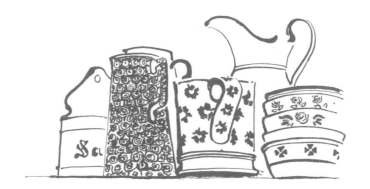

*delicious*

# CURRIED PARSNIP AND LENTIL SOUP★

### INGREDIENTS

| |
|---|
| 50g/2oz butter |
| 1 large onion, peeled and chopped |
| 2 large parsnips, peeled and chopped |
| 1litre/1¾pts chicken or vegetable stock |
| 1 rounded tsp curry ½ powder |
| salt and freshly ground black pepper, to taste |
| 125g/4oz red lentils |
| 150ml/5fl oz single cream milk : quite thick. |
| paprika, to garnish |

STARCH

*This is a comforting and warming winter soup. Serve it very hot, with a sprinkling of paprika.*

Melt the butter in a heavy pan, and cook the chopped onion until soft. Add the parsnips, stock, curry powder, seasoning, and lentils. Cover the pan and simmer over a low heat until the parsnips and lentils are cooked (30–45 minutes). Remove from the heat, and process or liquidize until smooth. (Don't worry if there are little lumps of parsnip left – they give the soup a more interesting texture.) Return to the pan and reheat gently. Add the cream, and check the seasoning.

# SPRINGTIME MINESTRONE

### INGREDIENTS

| |
|---|
| 500g/1lb mixed young spring vegetables: baby courgettes, small new carrots, baby turnips, tiny new potatoes, fresh peas |
| 1tbs olive oil |
| 1 nut of butter |
| 1 medium onion |
| 125g/4oz brown rice, well washed |
| 900ml/1½pts vegetable broth |
| a few leaves of fresh mint |
| salt and pepper |
| 2tbs fresh chopped parsley, to garnish |

STARCH

Clean all the vegetables. Finely slice the carrots and courgettes. Shell the peas. Clean and dice the turnips and potatoes.

Heat the oil and butter in a thick saucepan. Sweat the chopped onion in the oil, add all the other vegetables, and turn them until they glisten. Add the rice, and turn it over once or twice. Add the stock and the mint leaves, finely chopped. Bring to the boil, turn down the heat, and simmer, covered, until all the vegetables are cooked – about half an hour. Season the soup with salt and pepper to taste, and serve sprinkled with the parsley.

# RICE, ARTICHOKE, AND POTATO MINESTRONE

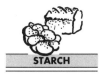

STARCH

Clean the artichokes (as on p.54), removing the tough outer leaves and tips. Slice them thinly. Scrub the potatoes and cut them into chunks. Melt the butter in a heavy pan, and turn the artichokes and potato pieces in it, until they start to take on a little colour. Sprinkle the flour over them, and turn around a little longer, stirring. Pour the stock over them, season, and bring to the boil. Cook for 10–15 minutes. Add the rice, and continue cooking until the rice is cooked through. Sprinkle with the parsley and serve immediately.

| INGREDIENTS |
| --- |
| 2 small globe artichokes |
| 2 medium potatoes |
| 1tbs butter |
| 1tsp wholewheat flour |
| 1.5litres/2¾pts light vegetable stock |
| 200g/7oz long-grain brown rice, well washed |
| salt and pepper |
| a bunch of fresh parsley, finely chopped |

# RICE AND LEEK MINESTRONE

STARCH

Clean and finely slice the leeks, including some of the green part. Heat the butter and oil in a heavy pan, add the leeks and onion, and let them fry gently until translucent. Add the rice and stir about until glistening with oil. Pour in the stock, season to taste, cover, and simmer for about an hour over a very low heat. Serve sprinkled with plenty of chopped parsley.

| INGREDIENTS |
| --- |
| 3 fine fat leeks |
| 25g/1oz butter |
| 1tbs olive oil |
| 1 large onion, finely chopped |
| 175g/6oz brown rice, well washed |
| 900ml/1½pt vegetable broth |
| salt and pepper |
| 2tbs chopped fresh parsley, to garnish |

## LETTUCE AND PEA SOUP

### INGREDIENTS

| |
|---|
| 50g/2oz butter |
| 1 large leek, trimmed and sliced |
| 2 medium potatoes, peeled and chopped |
| 375g/12oz lettuce leaves, washed and torn into pieces |
| 600ml/1pt vegetable stock |
| salt and freshly ground pepper |
| 125g/4oz fresh peas (frozen *petits pois* will do, if necessary) |
| freshly chopped parsley |

*This is a useful recipe for using up a garden glut of lettuces. Even "bolted" ones will do.*

Heat the butter in a large pan, and cook the leek, potatoes, and lettuce gently for about 5 minutes, turning them around in the hot butter. Add the stock, season to taste, and bring to the boil. Simmer gently for 20–30 minutes. Add the peas about halfway through the cooking time. Blend or process until smooth, then return to a clean pan, reheat, and check the seasoning. Serve with a sprinkling of chopped parsley.

STARCH

✓ SWEETCORN CHOWDER  *Yummy    Lewis's ✓✗    Heather No*

### INGREDIENTS

| |
|---|
| 1tbs olive oil |
| 2 onions, chopped |
| 2 sticks celery, chopped |
| 2 carrots, chopped |
| 1 medium potato, diced |
| 900ml/1½pts vegetable stock |
| 500g/1lb sweet corn – you can use frozen |
| a small bunch of fresh parsley, stalks trimmed off |
| salt and pepper |
| 1tbs single cream |

Heat the oil in a heavy pan, and cook the onions in it until just translucent. Add the celery, carrots, and potato, and turn around in the hot oil. Pour in the stock, bring to the boil, and simmer, covered, until the vegetables are done. Add the sweet corn, and continue simmering until it is soft. Season, add the parsley, then put through a food mouli if you have one, or blend or process – but only briefly: this should be a thick, rich soup full of texture with corn kernels still visible in it, rather than a purée. Just before serving, season and stir in the cream.

STARCH

# EGG DISHES FOR PROTEIN MEALS

## RUSTIC FRITTATA

**PROTEIN**

*A frittata is an Italian version of the omelette: a more substantial dish, thick enough to slice, with various herbs and vegetables added, and served cold as often as hot. Here are 3 different versions.*

Finely slice the spring onions, and let them soften gently in a little olive oil. Add the peas and the cleaned and sliced mushrooms. Mix and cook over very low heat for 15 minutes, stirring often. Drain and slice the artichoke hearts. Beat the eggs, season, and add the spring onions, mushrooms, artichokes, peas, and parsley. Heat the remaining oil in a non-stick pan, turn in the mixture, and cook the *frittata* over a very low heat. When the underside is done, slide the *frittata* out on to a plate. Add a little more oil to the pan and heat it. Return the *frittata* to the pan, the other way up. Cook the *frittata* gently for a few more minutes.

| INGREDIENTS |
| --- |
| 6–8 spring onions |
| 2–3tbs olive oil |
| 150g/5oz peas – fresh or frozen |
| 3–4 mushrooms |
| 125g/4oz artichoke hearts bottled in oil (most delicatessens sell these) |
| 5 eggs |
| salt and pepper |
| 1tbs fresh parsley, finely chopped |

## COURGETTE FRITTATA

**PROTEIN**

Start preparing this dish in the morning. Clean the courgettes, and slice them thinly. Heat 2tbs of olive oil – you may need more than this – in a frying-pan, and fry the courgettes, a few at a time. As they are ready, lift them out on to a plate with a slotted spoon. Clean the frying-pan, and add 1tbs of olive oil. Add the peeled and sliced garlic, white wine vinegar, a little pepper, and salt. Bring it to the boil, then pour it over the courgettes, and leave to marinate all day.

When you're ready to make the *frittata*, beat the eggs, add the courgettes – well drained – and season with pepper and salt. Heat a tbs of olive oil in a non-stick pan, add the egg mixture, and cook as explained above.

| INGREDIENTS |
| --- |
| 4 medium courgettes |
| 4tbs olive oil |
| 2 cloves garlic |
| 1 wineglass white wine vinegar |
| salt and pepper |
| 5 eggs |

# FRITTATA PROVENÇALE

### INGREDIENTS

| |
|---|
| 1 large aubergine |
| 1 red pepper |
| 1 clove garlic |
| 4tbs olive oil |
| 25g/1oz butter |
| 5 eggs |
| 2tbs grated parmesan cheese |
| 1tbs finely chopped parsley |
| salt and pepper |

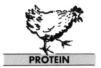

**PROTEIN**

Wash the aubergine, top and tail it, and slice into thin slices. Salt and leave to drain in a colander for half an hour. Meanwhile, turn the pepper under a hot grill or over a flame until the skin is charred and blistered. Wash off all the bits under cold running water, cut open, remove the seeds, and cut into strips. Drain and blot dry the aubergine slices, and chop the garlic. Heat the oil in a frying-pan. Add the garlic, but remove it when it has taken on colour. Add the aubergine slices, and fry until well browned on both sides. Drain them on kitchen paper. Beat the eggs with the cheese. Add the chopped parsley, the red pepper strips, and a little freshly ground pepper. Clean the pan, heat up 1tbs of oil and the butter, put in half the aubergine slices, and pour the egg mixture over them. Put the rest of the aubergine slices on top, and cook as described in the first *frittata* recipe, opposite.

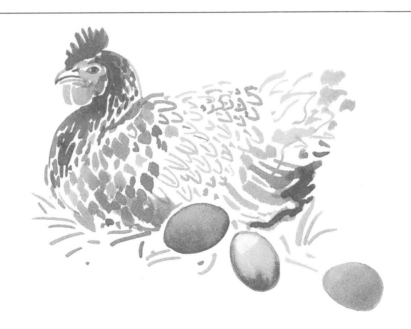

# EGGS BAKED IN TOMATOES

**PROTEIN**

Heat the oven to 180°C/350°F/gas 4. Wash the tomatoes, slice off a wide lid at the top of each one, and scrape out most of the flesh, taking care not to damage the skins. Put the tomato shells on a greased baking dish, and bake for about 10 minutes. Mix 3tbs of chopped-up tomato flesh with the chopped parsley, and season. Put a spoonful in each tomato, and crack an egg over the filling. Top with a spoonful of the grated cheese, and return to the oven for 10–15 minutes.

| INGREDIENTS |
| --- |
| 4 beef tomatoes |
| 4 eggs |
| 2tbs grated cheddar cheese |
| 1tbs parsley, chopped |
| salt and pepper |

# SCRAMBLED EGGS WITH MUSHROOMS★

*If you can't imagine scrambled eggs without that piece of toast, try any of these variations. Serve with a salad and a green vegetable.*

**PROTEIN**

Clean the mushrooms and chop into fairly small pieces. Clean and finely chop the onion and the garlic. Heat the oil in a frying-pan with a little butter, and fry the onions and garlic gently until they begin to take on colour. Remove, and add the mushrooms to the pan. Season them and fry briskly for 10–15 minutes, turning them over often.

Beat the eggs. Season. Add the chopped chives and pour over the mushrooms. Stir lightly with a wooden spoon or spatula until the eggs are set.

| INGREDIENTS |
| --- |
| 250g/8oz mushrooms |
| 2–3 spring onions |
| 2 cloves garlic |
| 2tbs olive oil |
| butter |
| 1 bunch of fresh parsley |
| 6 eggs |
| salt and pepper |
| chives |

## SCRAMBLED EGGS WITH PEPPERS AND TOMATOES★

### INGREDIENTS

| |
|---|
| 2 yellow peppers |
| 2tbs oil |
| 1 onion, finely chopped |
| 1 clove garlic, finely chopped |
| 2–3 big tomatoes, skinned and chopped (or you can use a small can of whole peeled tomatoes) |
| salt and pepper |
| a pinch of oregano |
| 5 eggs |
| 75g/3oz emmenthal cheese, cubed |
| 2tbs butter |
| plenty of fresh chopped parsley |

PROTEIN

Wash and clean the peppers, removing the white ribs and the seeds, and slice into thin strips. Heat the oil in a pan and add the onion and garlic. Let them cook for a minute or so, then add the chopped tomatoes, season them, and add the oregano and the strips of pepper. Cook over a fairly high heat for a few minutes, stirring often, then take off the heat and keep warm.

Beat the eggs in a bowl, add the cheese cubes, and season lightly. Heat the butter in a non-stick pan, pour in the egg mixture, stir with a fork and, when the eggs are creamy and set, pour the pepper and tomato mixture over the top. Sprinkle with the parsley and serve.

## SCRAMBLED EGGS WITH RICOTTA★

### INGREDIENTS

| |
|---|
| a good bunch of fresh mixed herbs – basil, mint, parsley, and chervil |
| 6 eggs |
| salt and pepper |
| 125g/4oz ricotta or other smooth cream cheese |
| 2tbs milk |
| 50g/2oz butter |
| watercress, to garnish |

PROTEIN

Finely chop the herbs – there should be a good 2tbs – and add to the well-beaten eggs. Season lightly. Beat the ricotta with the milk to a smooth paste, add the beaten eggs and herbs, and mix well. Heat the butter in a non-stick pan, add the eggs, and stir briskly with a wooden spoon until they are set to the point you like. Serve with sprigs of watercress, and a tossed green salad.

## OMELETTE ARNOLD BENNETT★

**PROTEIN**

*This quantity makes enough for 2 people: making it for more people at a time can be tricky.*

Heat half the butter in a pan. Take off the heat, and add the fish, the cream, and 1tbs of the cheese. Season. Add the fish mixture to the eggs, and set the grill to red hot.

Melt the rest of the butter in an omelette pan, and add the fish and egg mixture. Cook fairly quickly until it is beginning to set. Sprinkle the rest of the cheese over the top, and grill until the cheese bubbles. Sprinkle with the parsley and serve.

| INGREDIENTS |
| --- |
| 50g/2oz butter |
| 125g/4oz smoked haddock, cooked and flaked |
| 2tbs double cream |
| 2tbs grated parmesan cheese |
| salt and pepper |
| 3 eggs, well beaten |
| chopped fresh parsley |

## HARD-BOILED EGGS WITH TUNA AND GARLIC MAYONNAISE★

**PROTEIN**

Hard-boil the eggs, shell, and halve them. Flake the tuna into a shallow dish. Arrange the halved eggs on top, and spoon over the mayonnaise. Sprinkle a little paprika over them.

This dish can also make a filling starter.

| INGREDIENTS |
| --- |
| 4 eggs |
| 200g/7oz can of tuna |
| 4tbs Garlic Mayonnaise (p.144) |
| paprika |

# EGG DISH FOR A STARCH MEAL

## BAKED EGGS WITH SPINACH AND MUSHROOMS

### INGREDIENTS

| |
|---|
| 1kg/2lb fresh spinach or 500g/1lb frozen |
| a nut of butter |
| a pinch of nutmeg |
| salt and pepper |
| 2–3tbs olive oil |
| 250g/8oz mushrooms, cleaned and diced |
| 1 clove garlic, finely chopped |
| 4 egg yolks |
| 4tbs sour cream |

STARCH

Cook the spinach (as described p.62), drain, and chop very finely with a knife, or process briefly in the blender. (Aim to achieve a rough texture rather than a smooth purée.)

Add the butter, and stir it into the spinach. Season with nutmeg, pepper, and a very little salt. Keep to one side. Heat the oven to 200°C/400°F/gas 6.

Heat the oil in a frying-pan, and add the mushrooms and garlic. Cook until the mushrooms start to colour. Remove the mushrooms with a slotted spoon, and combine with the spinach purée. Grease 4 small, ovenproof cocottes. Make 4 rings in them of the spinach-mushroom mixture, put an egg yolk in the middle of each, and bake for 10–15 minutes, until the yolks are well set. Pour 1tbs of sour cream around each yolk before serving.

This dish can also be cooked in a shallow, ovenproof casserole, putting all the spinach-mushroom mixture in, and making 4 hollows for the egg yolks.

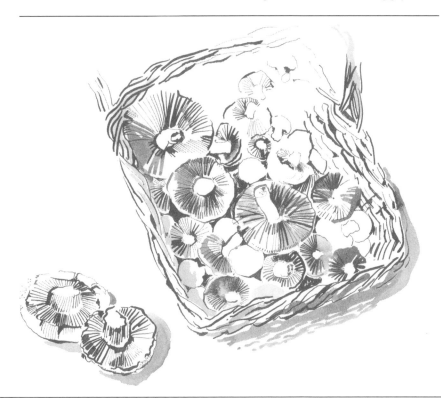

# FISH DISHES FOR PROTEIN MEALS

## FISH IN A FIERY SAUCE

**PROTEIN**

*This is fast and easy to prepare. The pale blandness of the fish contrasts dramatically with the hot, deep red sauce.*

Wash the fish, remove the skin, pat dry, and paint with oil and the juice of a lemon. Season with salt and freshly ground pepper.

To make the sauce, heat the oil in a pan, and fry the garlic until just translucent. Add the can of tomatoes, chop them up a bit, and allow to cook gently for a few minutes. Then add the wine, the seasoning, the herbs, and as much chilli as you desire (remember – a little goes a long way). Heat together gently, and let the sauce simmer for 10–15 minutes. The sauce can be made in advance and reheated when you're ready.

Heat the grill, put the fish steaks under it, and grill until they are cooked right through.

Serve with the hot sauce on the side, and a sharp, tossed green salad.

| INGREDIENTS |
| --- |
| **4 fish steaks or slices of firm-fleshed white fish** |
| **olive oil** |
| **juice of 1 lemon** |
| **salt and pepper** |
| **For the sauce:** |
| **2tbs olive oil** |
| **3 or 4 fat cloves garlic, finely chopped** |
| **425g/14oz can tomatoes** |
| **a little red or white wine, or water** |
| **salt and freshly ground pepper** |
| **a pinch of dried oregano** |
| **a pinch of dried thyme** |
| **chilli powder or flakes** |

## ORANGE-MARINATED MACKEREL

**PROTEIN**

Make 3 slits in each mackerel. Place in a shallow baking dish. Mix together the yogurt, orange rind, and ginger, and spoon over the fish. Leave for 2–3 hours. Heat the oven to 180°C/350°F/gas 4. Bake for 25–30 minutes.

| INGREDIENTS |
| --- |
| **4 mackerel, cleaned** |
| **300ml/½pt plain yogurt** |
| **grated rind of 1 well-scrubbed orange** |
| **1tsp grated fresh ginger** |

## SALMON WITH ORANGE SAUCE★

### INGREDIENTS

| |
| --- |
| **4 salmon steaks, each about 150g/5oz** |
| **1½tsp peppercorns** |
| **1½tsp coriander seeds** |
| **1tbs olive oil** |
| **15g/½oz unsalted butter** |
| **120ml/4fl oz fresh orange juice** |
| **120ml/4fl oz fish stock or white wine** |
| **120ml/4fl oz single cream** |
| **salt and pepper** |
| **To garnish:** |
| **fresh coriander or parsley sprigs** |
| **a little grated orange rind** |

Try to persuade the fishmonger to skin the steaks for you. Otherwise, trim them off with a sharp paring knife, together with any odd bones. Separate the skinned steaks into 2 halves. Grind the peppercorns and coriander seeds together. Toss the salmon pieces in this mixture. Heat the oil and butter in a frying-pan, and cook the salmon pieces over a gentle heat for about 10 minutes, turning occasionally until they are light golden in colour. Remove from the pan and keep warm.

Add the orange juice and fish stock or white wine to the pan. Bring to the boil, scraping up all the bits. Stir in the cream, and continue boiling until the liquid reduces to a thin sauce. Strain. Arrange the pieces of fish on a hot serving plate, and pour the sauce over them. Garnish with the fresh coriander or parsley, and the grated orange rind.

## MUSTARD-MARINATED SALMON

### INGREDIENTS

| |
| --- |
| **For the marinade:** |
| **4tbs olive oil** |
| **4tbs dry white wine** |
| **4tbs lemon juice** |
| **2tbs Dijon mustard** |
| **2tbs onion, finely chopped** |
| **salt and pepper** |
| **4 salmon steaks, each about 175g/6oz** |
| **To garnish:** |
| **slices of lemon** |
| **sprigs of watercress** |

Shake the marinade ingredients in a screw-top jar. Pour into a large, shallow dish. Add the salmon steaks and turn so that they are well coated with the marinade. Put in the refrigerator or a cool place for about 3 hours, turning them over once.

Heat the grill. Grease the grill rack with a little oil, then put the salmon steaks on it. Brush each steak with some of the marinade, and grill for about 4 minutes on each side.

# LEMON-MARINATED SARDINES

**PROTEIN**

Cut the sardines open and gut them, chop off the heads, and remove the backbones. (This sounds messy and difficult but you'll find you become practised quite quickly.) Wash the sardines thoroughly and blot dry on kitchen paper.

Heat the grill to red hot, and lay the sardines flat in the grill pan (you'll probably have to cook them in 2 batches). Brush the sardines with 2tbs of the olive oil, and grill on both sides until they are just changing colour – perhaps a minute in all.

Take the sardines out and arrange them in a shallow white oval dish. Put the grill pan over a low flame, and add the finely chopped garlic and the white wine. Bring to the boil, allow to bubble and reduce a little, then add the lemon juice and the freshly ground black pepper. Pour the sauce over the sardines, and sprinkle with the parsley and the grated rind. Cover with a damp cloth or clingfilm, and leave to chill for a couple of hours.

Serve with a refreshing Cucumber Salad (p.130).

### INGREDIENTS

| |
|---|
| 16–20 sardines |
| 3tbs olive oil |
| 2 cloves garlic, very finely chopped |
| 2tbs white wine |
| juice and grated rind of 1 lemon |
| freshly ground black pepper |
| 2tbs fresh parsley, chopped |

# SALT-FRIED SARDINES

**PROTEIN**

*A fishmonger in the marvellous waterfront market at Honfleur suggested this way of cooking the sea-fresh, bright sardines he sold us. It is simplicity itself. Fresh anchovies can be cooked in the same way.*

Clean the sardines (an obliging fishmonger will show you how, if in doubt). Wash them and pat dry. Heat a heavy iron or stainless steel frying-pan to near red-hot, put in 2–3 handfuls of sea salt, and let it heat through: a fairly noisy business. Lay your sardines on the salt, and fry over a high heat until they are beautifully browned on both sides. Brush off the salt and serve.

### INGREDIENTS

| |
|---|
| 5–6 sardines per person |
| sea salt |

## FISHBURGERS

### INGREDIENTS

**500g/1lb cooked white fish, or canned (drain off any oil or brine)**

**1 egg, well beaten**

**2tbs wheatgerm**

**2–3 spring onions, cleaned, trimmed, and very finely chopped (include some of the green part)**

**salt and pepper**

**oil, for frying**

**1 lemon, quartered, to garnish**

Flake the fish, and mix all the ingredients very thoroughly. Alternatively, put them in a blender or food processor, and process very briefly. Form the mixture into burgers, dust with more wheatgerm, and sauté for 2–3 minutes on each side. Serve with a quarter of lemon for each helping.

**PROTEIN**

## FISH WITH RED ONIONS

### INGREDIENTS

**750g/1½lbs fillets of any flat fish**

**salt and pepper**

**mixed herbs**

**2 red onions, sliced**

**4tbs red wine**

**juice and zest of 1 lemon**

**1tbs olive oil**

**1tsp butter**

**fresh tarragon, to garnish**

Wash, dry, and season the fish. Sprinkle with the mixed herbs and set aside. Put the onion, wine, and lemon juice and zest, into an ovenproof dish with a cover. Cook over a medium heat, stirring occasionally until soft. Heat the oil and butter in a large frying-pan, and fry the fish until just golden, 3–4 minutes on each side. Arrange a bed of onion on each plate, place the fillets on top, and garnish with the fresh tarragon.

**PROTEIN**

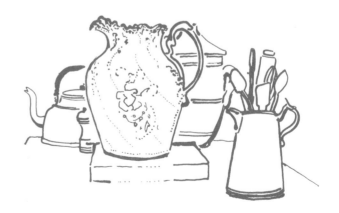

# FISH SALADS

Fish with its mild delicate flavour, when poached, steamed, or baked and served cold, dressed with a tangy or creamy sauce, is a lovely dish for a weekend meal, or for a summer buffet party. Salmon, whiting, or any firm-fleshed white fish are all good candidates for this treatment. Frozen fish, frankly, won't do: its limp, woolly texture won't stand up to this gourmet treatment. Here is a basic recipe for cooking fish, and 3 sauces to serve with it.

## COLD POACHED FISH

**PROTEIN**

Put the water in a pan and add all the other ingredients. Bring to the boil, and simmer for 30 minutes. Then strain and let cool. When the liquid is cold, put your fish in it – there should be just enough liquid to cover it, don't use any more. Bring to the boil over a very gentle heat. When the liquid boils, let it bubble gently for 2–3 minutes, then remove from the heat. Let the fish cool in the liquid. It should be cooked through, but still firm. Skin and bone it, if necessary. Arrange on a large dish, and serve with one of the following 3 sauces.

| INGREDIENTS |
|---|
| **750g/1½lbs any firm white fish** |
| **For the court bouillon:** |
| **1 litre/1¾pt water** |
| **300ml/½pt dry white wine** |
| **2tbs white wine vinegar or apple vinegar** |
| **10 peppercorns** |
| **1 carrot, cleaned and sliced** |
| **1 onion, cleaned and sliced** |
| **1 sprig of thyme** |

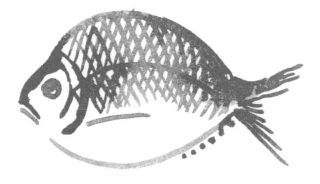

## GREEN MAYONNAISE

### INGREDIENTS

| 1 bunch of watercress |
| 1 bunch of parsley |
| some spinach leaves |
| chives, tarragon, chervil, as available |
| 6–8tbs Mayonnaise |

Clean the leaves, and strip from the stalks. Put the herbs in a pan with 2–3 tbs of water and simmer for 5 minutes. (Add more water if necessary.) Put the mixture in a blender, and stir the resulting green cream into a bowl of Mayonnaise (p.144).

PROTEIN

## LEMON AND YOGURT SAUCE

### INGREDIENTS

| 150g/5oz thick plain yogurt |
| 2tbs lemon juice |
| grated rind of 1 well-scrubbed lemon |
| 3tbs grated onion |
| 2tbs finely chopped fresh parsley |
| 1tsp Dijon mustard |
| salt and pepper |

Combine all the ingredients, and season to taste. Sour cream can be used instead of yogurt.

PROTEIN

## FRESH TOMATO SAUCE

### INGREDIENTS

| 1 small onion, finely chopped |
| 3–4 big, ripe tomatoes, skinned and chopped |
| 2 cloves garlic |
| 1tbs olive oil |
| sprigs of parsley, stalks removed |
| 5–6 basil leaves |
| ½ red pepper, deseeded and finely diced |
| 2 stalks of celery, very finely diced |
| salt and pepper |

Put the onion, tomatoes, garlic, olive oil, and herbs in a blender or food processor. Blend very briefly – the result shouldn't be too smooth. Stir in the red pepper and celery. Season to taste. Chill for half an hour before serving.

PROTEIN

# FISH WITH A SPICED YOGURT CRUST

**PROTEIN**

Clean the fish pieces, blot them dry, and put them in a shallow, fireproof dish. Put all the other ingredients in a blender or food processor, and process until well mixed. Cover the fish with the mixture, and leave for 2–3 hours, for the flavours to marry with the fish. Heat the grill to red hot, and put the fish under it. Grill, basting regularly, until a crust forms on top.

| INGREDIENTS |
| --- |
| **4 pieces of firm-fleshed white fish, each weighing approx. 250g/8oz** |
| **300ml/10fl oz natural yogurt** |
| **1 medium onion, peeled and chopped** |
| **2 cloves garlic, skinned and crushed** |
| **3tbs coriander seeds** |
| **2tbs fresh mint, chopped** |
| **2tsp ground cumin** |
| **2tsp dried dill** |
| **2tsp paprika** |
| **1 good grating of nutmeg** |
| **2tbs fresh parsley, chopped** |

# FISH WITH GINGER AND SPRING ONIONS

**PROTEIN**

Heat the oven to 180°C/350°F/gas 4. Put a large sheet of baking foil over a large ovenproof dish. Lightly oil the foil and spread the onions over it. Sprinkle on the ginger, coriander, and freshly ground black pepper. Place the fish on top and close up the foil, pinching the edges together to form a loose parcel. Bake the fish for 30 minutes.

| INGREDIENTS |
| --- |
| **1tbs olive oil** |
| **8 spring onions, finely sliced lengthways** |
| **1 small piece of fresh ginger root, peeled and grated** |
| **1tbs fresh chopped coriander leaves** |
| **freshly ground black pepper** |
| **4 150g/5oz fish steaks – any firm-fleshed white fish will do** |

# POACHED TROUT WITH WATERCRESS AND MUSHROOM STUFFING

**PROTEIN**

## INGREDIENTS

**4 pink rainbow trout, each weighing approx. 350g/12oz, cleaned and boned**

**For the stuffing:**

**a bunch of watercress**

**1 medium onion, peeled and finely chopped**

**25g/1oz butter**

**50g/2oz mushrooms, cleaned and sliced**

**grated rind of 2 well-scrubbed lemons**

**2tsp lemon juice**

**2tsp horseradish sauce**

**600ml/1pt fish stock, or half fish stock and half white wine or dry cider**

**50g/2oz butter**

**3tbs single cream**

**salt and freshly ground pepper**

Trim the watercress, then wash and finely chop it, reserving a few sprigs for garnishing. Fry the onion in the butter until soft, add the watercress, and stir well. Remove from the heat and add the rest of the stuffing ingredients. Put on one side while you prepare the trout.

Heat the oven to 190°C/375°F/gas 5. Wash and dry the fish, then sprinkle a little salt and pepper inside. Pack the stuffing inside, and close tightly. Choose a baking dish the trout will just fit into. Pour in the stock – it should just cover the fish – and lemon juice. Cover with foil and bake for about 30 minutes, or until the fish is done. Drain off the cooking liquid, lower the oven temperature, and put the fish back in the oven to keep it hot. Put the fishy liquid in a saucepan, and boil briskly to reduce by about half. Whisk in the butter, check the seasoning, and add the cream. Pour the liquid over the trout, garnish with the watercress, and serve.

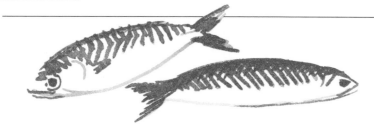

# Meat, Game, and Poultry for Protein Meals

## RABBIT WITH ANCHOVY SAUCE

**PROTEIN**

Wash and dry the rabbit pieces. Put them in a bowl with the chopped onion, the cleaned and chopped carrot, the sliced celery, parsley, bay leaf, and a sprinkling of *fines herbes*. Add a little sea salt. Pour over the red wine, and leave to marinate for 4–5 hours. Then take out and dry the rabbit pieces.

Heat the oil in a casserole, and add the rabbit. Let it brown on all sides, then sprinkle with the potato flour. Add the herbs, and pour in the wine drained from the marinade. Let the wine bubble and reduce, then add a glass or two of vegetable stock – enough to make a good thick sauce. Lower the heat, and cover the casserole. Cook until the rabbit is tender – about an hour.

When it is ready, transfer the rabbit to another casserole and keep warm. Add a tablespoon or so of hot water to the cooking pan, scrape up all the juices, and add to the rabbit. Finely chop the anchovy fillets, add the parsley, garlic, a little pepper, vinegar, and the white wine. Mix well, and add to the rabbit. Cover and simmer over a very low heat for another 5 minutes.

### INGREDIENTS

| |
|---|
| 1 large rabbit, jointed, or about 750g/1½lb rabbit pieces |
| 1 large onion |
| 2 or 3 stalks of celery |
| 2 carrots |
| parsley |
| 1 small bay leaf |
| *fines herbes* |
| salt |
| 1 generous glass of red wine |
| 2tbs olive oil |
| 1tsp potato flour |
| **For the anchovy sauce:** |
| 2–3 fillets of anchovy, rinsed and soaked in water for about an hour |
| 1tbs finely chopped parsley |
| freshly ground pepper |
| 1 clove garlic, very finely chopped |
| 1tbs cider or white wine vinegar |
| 2tbs white wine |

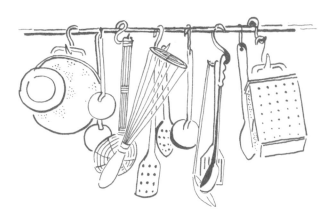

# ROSALIND'S RABBIT WITH PRUNES

### INGREDIENTS

| |
|---|
| 1 rabbit, cut into serving pieces |
| 300ml/½pt red wine, for marinade |
| 4 carrots, cleaned and sliced |
| 1 large onion, sliced |
| 2 bay leaves |
| salt and pepper |
| 2tbs butter |
| 2tbs olive oil |
| 200g/7oz dried prunes |
| 1–2tbs redcurrant jelly |

PROTEIN

*At their house Il Casino which she and her husband rebuilt from a ruin deep in a tranquil valley, Ros Colley serves this typically Tuscan dish to appreciative guests.*

Wash the rabbit pieces, blot dry, and put into a china bowl with the red wine, carrots, onions, bay leaves, salt, and pepper. Marinate for 24 hours. Wash the prunes and put them to soak in 300ml/½pint boiling water.

Drain, and pat dry, reserving the marinade. Heat the oil and butter in a pan, and sauté the rabbit pieces until coloured. Add the marinade liquid: there should be enough to cover, but top up with more wine if necessary, or some of the prune juice. Add the soaked prunes, bring to the boil, skim, and simmer until tender – about 45 minutes. Arrange the rabbit pieces and prunes on a serving dish. Reduce the sauce over a high heat, correct the seasoning, and blend the jelly into the sauce. Pour over the rabbit pieces and serve.

A purée of turnips and a watercress salad go well with this dish.

# RABBIT WITH BLACK OLIVES

### INGREDIENTS

| |
|---|
| 1kg/2lb rabbit, cut into pieces |
| 4tbs olive oil |
| 1tbs butter |
| 2 cloves garlic |
| sprigs of fresh thyme |
| 1 large onion, finely chopped |
| salt and pepper |
| 1 glass of dry white wine |
| vegetable stock or water |
| 12 stoned black olives |

PROTEIN

Wash and dry the rabbit pieces. Heat the oil and the butter in a casserole, and add the chopped garlic and the sprigs of thyme. Leave them for a minute or so to diffuse their aromas into the oil. Add the rabbit, sauté until it is browned on all sides, add the onion, and season. Pour in the wine, and raise the heat. Let the liquid bubble and reduce for a few minutes, then turn the heat down. Add a couple of tablespoons of stock, cover, and cook over a low flame – barely a simmer – for about an hour, or until the rabbit is tender. (This is a dish that can be kept warm for at least half an hour, so you can allow plenty of time for cooking.) Five minutes before serving, add the black olives.

# GRILLED SPICED CHICKEN

PROTEIN

*This is an easy recipe to make which takes minutes to prepare. It can be eaten hot, perhaps with one of the vegetable casseroles or purées, or cold with a sharp, tangy salad.*

Skin the chicken breasts, then wash and dry them. Chop the onion, and crush the garlic. Put them in a bowl with the yogurt. Heat the coriander and cumin seeds – toss them in a frying-pan over a low heat for a minute or so – then crush and add to the yogurt, together with the paprika and chilli. Mix well. Put the chicken in a bowl, pour over the spicy yogurt mixture, and leave to marinate for at least a couple of hours.

Heat the grill to maximum. Grill the chicken pieces until cooked – about 25 minutes – basting them with the marinade and turning them occasionally.

| INGREDIENTS |
| --- |
| 500g/1lb boneless chicken breasts |
| 1 small onion |
| 2 cloves garlic |
| 150g/5oz natural yogurt |
| 1tsp coriander seeds |
| 1tsp cumin seeds |
| 1tsp paprika |
| ½tsp chilli powder |
| sea salt |

# RED-HOT CHICKEN

PROTEIN

Clean and slice the sweet peppers, removing all the seeds. Wash and dry the chilli, then slice under cold running water, removing all the fiery seeds. Chop the onion finely. Cook the peppers, chilli, and onion in boiling water until they are tender, then blend in a food processor with the oil and lemon juice. Skin the chicken pieces, wash and wipe dry, then put them in a dish and pour the sauce over them. Leave overnight – or all day long.

Grill the chicken pieces until they are done, basting with the fiery sauce. You can use chilli powder or flakes instead – add them to the puréed sauce and reheat to absorb the flavours.

Serve with a cucumber salad, a slice of lemon, and crisp lettuce leaves.

| INGREDIENTS |
| --- |
| 2 sweet red peppers |
| 1 red chilli – or ½tsp chilli flakes |
| 1 medium onion |
| 2–3tbs olive oil |
| juice of 1 lemon |
| 4 chicken breasts or thighs, or 8 drumsticks, according to preference |

# TANGERINE CHICKEN PARCELS

### INGREDIENTS

| |
|---|
| 2 whole chicken breasts |
| 3 tangerines or seedless clementines, plus the grated rind of 2 of them (scrub well) |
| 3tbs olive oil |
| salt and pepper |
| 4 small sprigs of rosemary |
| 4 small sprigs of parsley |
| 4 slices of lemon |

Preheat the oven to 200°C/400°F/gas 6. Wipe the chicken breasts clean, halve them, beat flat, and put each one on a 30cm/12in square of baking foil. Juice the tangerines, add to the olive oil with salt and pepper, and mix well. Lay a sprig of each herb and a slice of lemon on the chicken breasts, with a good pinch of the grated tangerine rind. Pour over the liquid and close the parcels by gathering up the edges of the foil, and folding them together so that no liquid can escape.

Put the parcels in the oven and bake for 35 minutes. Serve the parcels on a big dish, then give each person their own parcel.

# COLD CHICKEN ROTHSCHILD WITH GRAPES AND LEMON AND TARRAGON SAUCE★

### INGREDIENTS

| |
|---|
| 1.5kg/3lb chicken |
| 1 carrot, peeled and sliced |
| 1 stick of celery, cleaned and sliced |
| 2 bay leaves |
| a few peppercorns |
| 1 small onion, skinned and halved |
| 50ml/2fl oz dry white wine |
| juice and grated rind of 1 well-scrubbed lemon |
| 150ml/5oz fresh whipping cream |
| 1tbs clear honey |
| 2 level tbs fresh tarragon, finely chopped |
| 250g/8oz seedless white grapes, well washed |
| mixed green lettuce leaves |
| paprika |

Put the chicken in a large pan with enough water to just cover it. Add the carrot, celery, bay leaves, peppercorns, and onion. Poach gently until cooked – about an hour. Remove the chicken from the pan, and set aside to cool. Strain the stock, and put about 300ml/¹⁄₂pt in a heavy-based saucepan. (Save the remaining stock for soups, etc.) Add the wine and the lemon juice, and boil rapidly, until reduced by about half. Set aside to cool.

When the chicken has cooled, remove the flesh from the bones, discarding the skin. Cut into small, even pieces, put in a bowl, and add the cream – whipped until it just holds its shape – the lemon rind, honey, seasoning, and tarragon. Fold in the reduced stock, amalgamate, and lastly, add the grapes. Chill thoroughly, and serve on a bed of lettuce, lightly dusted with paprika.

# CHICKEN WITH ONIONS

**PROTEIN**

Clean and wipe the chicken. Chop the onions finely. Heat the oil in a fireproof casserole big enough to take the chicken with room to spare, add the garlic, sage, and rosemary, and let them heat gently in the oil to release their aromatic flavours. Put in the chicken and brown lightly on all sides, for about 30 minutes. Remove the rosemary, sage, and garlic. Add the onions to the casserole and, as soon as they start to change colour, pour in the white wine. Allow to bubble and reduce a little. Turn down the heat, and cover the casserole. Cook until the chicken is done. (Golden juices should run clear when you pierce a thigh with a skewer.)

| INGREDIENTS |
| --- |
| 1 medium chicken |
| 500g/1lb onions |
| 3tbs olive oil |
| 2 cloves garlic |
| 2 leaves of sage |
| a sprig of rosemary |
| 1 glass dry white wine |
| salt and pepper |

# CURRIED CHICKEN WITH PEACHES

**PROTEIN**

*You can make 300ml/¹/₂pt nut milk, by infusing 4tbs ground almonds or dessicated coconut in 300ml/¹/₂pt boiling water for about an hour. Strain the liquid before use.*

Fry the chopped onion and garlic in the butter until soft. Stir in the curry powder, ginger, and cinnamon. Cook gently for a few minutes. Blend in the milk or nut milk, then stir in the chicken and seasoning. Bring to the boil, then lower the heat and simmer gently for about 30 minutes. Stir in the redcurrant jelly and sliced peaches. Cook gently for about 10 minutes, until heated through.

Serve with plain yogurt, perhaps with chopped cucumber added. This versatile dish can also be enjoyed cold with a salad.

| INGREDIENTS |
| --- |
| 1 medium onion, finely chopped |
| 1 clove garlic, crushed |
| 25g/1oz butter |
| 1 level tbs curry powder |
| ½tsp ground ginger |
| ½tsp ground cinnamon |
| 300ml/½pt milk or nut milk |
| 500g/1lb cooked chicken, chopped |
| salt and freshly ground pepper |
| 1tbs redcurrant jelly |
| 2 medium peaches (white-fleshed if possible), peeled and sliced |

# WELSH SALT DUCK

### INGREDIENTS

**1 large duck, about 2½kg/6lbs**

**125g/4oz coarse sea salt**

PROTEIN

*Elizabeth David describes this wonderful, startlingly simple recipe – which she herself adapted from an old Welsh cookery book – in her study of traditional English cooking,* Spices, Salt and Aromatics in the English Kitchen. *Served cold, the duck is tender and succulent, the perfect centrepiece for a festive summer lunch.*

"Buy your duck 3 days in advance. Place it in a deep dish and rub it all over with the salt. Repeat this process twice a day for 3 days. Keep the duck covered, and in a cool place. (Use the giblets at once for stock, and the liver for an omelette.)

"In the morning (for the following evening), first rinse off excess salt; then place the bird in a deep ovenproof dish. (I use a large, oval enamelled casserole, which will stand inside a baking tin.) Cover the duck with cold water. Put water also in the outer tin, then transfer to the centre of a very low oven, 150°C/300°F/gas 2. Cook uncovered for just 2 hours. Remove the duck from its liquid (which will be rather salty for use as stock) and leave the bird to cool."

Serve a sharp, fruity salad to accompany this dish: perhaps slices of oranges with watercress.

# TURKEY TONNATO

### INGREDIENTS

**2 carrots**

**1 celery stick**

**1 onion**

**1tbs white wine vinegar**

**2 turkey breasts**

**250g/8oz tuna, canned in oil**

**2tbs Mayonnaise (p.95)**

**2 fillets anchovy, soaked for a few minutes**

**1tbs capers**

**slices of lemon, to garnish**

PROTEIN

Bring plenty of salted water to the boil, then add the carrots, celery, and onion, cleaned and chopped, and the white wine vinegar. Let the stock boil for a few minutes, add the turkey, lower the heat, and leave to cook for about 45 minutes. Meanwhile, blend the tuna with the mayonnaise, anchovy fillets, capers, and enough oil to make a thick sauce. Season. Slice the turkey thinly – while it is still hot – arrange on a serving dish, and pour over the tuna sauce. This can be served hot or cold, garnished with lemon slices.

# TURKEY WITH ANCHOVY SAUCE

PROTEIN

*Turkey is not only economical: it's also impressively low in fats – a mere 1 per cent saturated fat in roast turkey compared to 3.8 in lean roast beef. If you only know turkey as the centrepiece of the Christmas feast, complete with bacon, sausages, stuffing, and all the trimmings, try these 2 recipes for cold turkey, each served with a piquant fishy sauce to contrast with the rather bland flavour of the meat. Either dish could star in a summer buffet.*

Bring plenty of salted water to the boil, add the carrot, celery, and onion, cleaned and chopped, and the white wine vinegar. Let the stock boil for a few minutes, then add the turkey, lower the heat, and leave to cook for about 45 minutes. Leave the turkey to cool in its broth. (Save this stock for soups.) Hard-boil the egg, shell, and chop it. Put the chopped egg in a blender with the anchovies – previously soaked for a few minutes – the parsley, seasoning, and enough oil to make a creamy sauce. Slice the turkey and serve covered with the sauce.

| INGREDIENTS |
| --- |
| 1 carrot |
| 1 celery stick |
| 1 onion |
| 1tbs white wine vinegar |
| 500g/1lb fresh, plump turkey breasts |
| 1 egg |
| 2 anchovy fillets |
| 2tbs parsley, finely chopped |
| olive oil |
| salt and pepper |

# STIR-FRIED TURKEY BREASTS WITH CELERY, WALNUTS, AND ORANGE

PROTEIN

Grate the rind from the well-scrubbed oranges, and peel them. Remove the white pith, and divide the flesh into segments. Reserve. Mix together the orange rind, the extra juice, the soya sauce, the sugar, the ginger, and the seasonings. Fry the onion and celery gently in 1tbs of the oil until they are soft. Use a wok, if possible; alternatively, use a large frying-pan. Remove from the pan with a slotted spoon, and add the remaining oil to the pan or wok. When hot, add the turkey strips and cook gently, stirring frequently, until the meat is cooked (about 10 minutes). The meat should be light brown in colour when it is cooked through.

Return the onion and celery to the pan with the turkey. Add the orange mixture, stir in the walnuts and the orange segments, and mix thoroughly. Stir gently until the ingredients are heated through.

| INGREDIENTS |
| --- |
| 2 oranges |
| 3tbs orange juice |
| 2tbs soya sauce |
| 1tbs soft brown sugar |
| ½tsp ground ginger |
| salt and freshly ground black pepper |
| 1 medium onion, cleaned and chopped |
| 4 sticks of celery, cleaned and chopped |
| 3tbs walnut or sesame oil |
| 600g/1¼lb turkey breast or escalopes, cut into strips |
| 125g/4oz broken walnuts |

# TURKEY BREASTS WITH LEMON AND WHITE WINE

### INGREDIENTS

**2 turkey breasts, each weighing 375g/12oz**

**2tbs olive oil**

**3–4 cloves garlic, finely chopped**

**125ml/4fl oz dry white wine**

**juice of ½ a lemon**

**salt and pepper**

PROTEIN

Wipe the turkey breasts clean. Cut them into small cubes. Heat the oil in a heavy pan, add the garlic, and let it just take on colour over a low flame. Take out the garlic, turn up the heat, and add the turkey cubes. Fry the cubes, turning them over 3 or 4 times so that they brown on all sides, then continue frying until they are cooked right through. Return the garlic to the pan, and turn up the heat. Add the wine, let it sizzle, and reduce to about half its original volume. Add the lemon juice, season, and serve.

# PHEASANT WITH APPLE, CELERY, AND CIDER

### INGREDIENTS

**2 medium-sized sweet eating apples**

**2 sticks of celery**

**1 medium onion**

**1 clove garlic**

**2tbs olive oil**

**2 hen pheasants**

**900ml/1½pt dry cider**

**1 bay leaf**

**1tsp juniper berries**

**salt and pepper**

PROTEIN

Preheat the oven to 180°C/350°F/gas 4. Wash, core, and chop the apples. Clean and slice the celery. Peel and finely chop the onion. Peel and chop the garlic. Heat the oil in a heavy, ovenproof casserole, big enough to hold the 2 birds and the vegetables. Sear the pheasants in the hot oil until they take on colour all over, and then put them to one side. Add the onions and garlic to the casserole – add a little more oil if necessary – and let them fry very gently until they are transparent. Then add the apples and the celery, and fry all the ingredients together for a couple of minutes.

Use half the mixture to stuff the 2 birds. Then return them to the casserole, add the rest of the apple-celery mixture, and pour in the cider. Let it come gently to the boil, and add the bay leaf and juniper berries. Season to taste, cover the casserole, and put in the oven to cook until the birds are tender – about an hour, depending on how well done you like them.

There should be plenty of thick sauce. If there is too much, strain off the liquid and reduce quickly in another pan, keeping the pheasants hot meanwhile.

# LAMB CHOP WITH TARRAGON AND CUCUMBER★

**PROTEIN**

Cut the cucumber into 8 sticks, sprinkle with salt, and leave in a colander for about 15 minutes, then rinse and drain. Heat the grill. Season the chops, and grill for about 5 minutes on each side. Remove and keep hot. Beat together the cream and egg yolks, then add the tarragon. Melt half the butter in a medium-sized pan, and cook the cucumber gently for about 5 minutes. Remove the cucumber (keep it warm). Add the cream and egg-yolk mixture to the buttery juices in the pan. Heat through gently but don't let the mixture boil. Arrange the chops and the cucumber on a warm dish, garnish with the tarragon sprigs, and serve the sauce separately.

| INGREDIENTS |
| --- |
| ½ a medium cucumber, peeled, cut in half, and deseeded |
| salt and freshly ground black pepper |
| 8 noisettes of lamb or neck cutlets |
| 150ml/5oz single cream |
| 2 egg yolks |
| 50g/2oz butter |
| 2tbs fresh tarragon, chopped |
| sprigs of fresh tarragon, to garnish |

# SALLY'S LAMB

**PROTEIN**

Preheat the oven to 180°C/350°F/gas 4. Trim all the surplus fat from the lamb. Heat 2tbs of the oil in a large, cast-iron casserole. Brown the lamb in the oil until sealed all over, turning it from side to side. Remove from the pan, add more of the oil if needed, with the garlic, onion, and seasoning, and sweat until transparent. Add the lentils and stir over a moderate heat for 5 minutes without letting the onions brown. Return the leg of lamb to the casserole, and add the wine, bay leaves, and bouquet garni. Cover and place in the preheated oven for 1½ hours. Add a little water during cooking if required. Remove the lamb from the pot and leave it to stand, covered with foil, for 10 minutes. Carve into chunks and serve on top of the lentils.

| INGREDIENTS |
| --- |
| 1 medium leg of lamb |
| 4tbs olive oil |
| 2 cloves garlic, chopped |
| 2 onions, sliced |
| 125/4oz green lentils |
| 300ml/½pt red wine |
| 2 bay leaves |
| 1 bouquet garni |
| salt and pepper |

# VEGETABLE DISHES FOR PROTEIN MEALS

## CAULIFLOWER TONNATO

### INGREDIENTS

| |
|---|
| **1 medium cauliflower, washed and trimmed** |
| **juice of 1 lemon** |
| **salt and freshly ground pepper** |
| **200g/7oz can of tuna in brine** |
| **4tbs Mayonnaise (p.144)** |
| **4tbs natural yogurt** |
| **1tbs capers** |
| **3 gherkins, finely chopped** |
| **3tbs chopped parsley** |

Cook the cauliflower whole in a pan with a little lemon juice, a pinch of salt, and enough boiling water to come halfway up the cauliflower. Cover the pan and simmer over a low heat until the cauliflower is just tender – about 10–15 minutes. Meanwhile, mix the rest of the ingredients together, including the remaining lemon juice. (Save 1tbs of the parsley for garnishing.) Heat the dish through in a bowl over a pan of gently simmering water. Season to taste.

Drain the cooked cauliflower and place in a warm, shallow serving dish. Spoon the warm tonnato sauce over the top and serve immediately, sprinkled with the rest of the parsley.

**PROTEIN**

## BAKED TOMATO GRATIN★

### INGREDIENTS

| |
|---|
| **4 beefsteak or 6 medium tomatoes** |
| **4 medium onions** |
| **200g/7oz emmenthal cheese** |
| **3 eggs** |
| **salt and pepper** |
| **175g/6oz single cream** |
| **butter** |
| **1 sprig of fresh basil, or 1tsp dried oregano** |

Heat the oven to 200°C/400°F/gas 6. Wash and slice the tomatoes. Skin and finely slice the onions. Grate the cheese. Beat the eggs with a little salt and pepper, and add the cream. Butter a fireproof casserole. Put a layer of the onions on the bottom, sprinkle a little of the cheese over them, top with a layer of the sliced tomatoes, and sprinkle with a little more cheese. Continue layering until all the vegetables are used up, topping with a layer of tomatoes. Scatter the finely chopped fresh basil – or the dried oregano – over the top, and pour over the cream and egg mixture. Put in the oven and bake for about 30 minutes.

**PROTEIN**

# RED AND YELLOW CASSEROLE★

**PROTEIN**

Wash the aubergine, and slice it finely. Put the slices in a colander, sprinkle with 1tbs of salt, and leave for about an hour, for the bitter juices to drain out. Clean the peppers, remove the seeds and fleshy bits from the insides, and slice into strips. Wash the courgettes and tomatoes, and slice them finely. Slice the onion finely. Skin and finely chop the garlic. Clean and chop the parsley and basil.

Heat the oven to 180°C/350°F/gas 4. Oil an ovenproof casserole. Rinse and blot dry the aubergine slices, and layer them over the bottom of the casserole. Season, sprinkle with some of the chopped herbs, and drizzle a little oil on top. Follow the aubergines with a layer of tomatoes, then the courgettes, then the onions and garlic, and finally the strips of pepper, seasoning each layer, and adding a little of the herbs and a touch of oil.

Cover with a piece of foil, and bake in the oven for 45 minutes. Then remove the foil, sprinkle the top with the grated cheese, and return to the oven until the cheese is melted and golden-brown.

| INGREDIENTS |
| --- |
| 1 aubergine |
| 1 large red pepper |
| 1 large yellow pepper |
| 2 courgettes |
| 2–3 tomatoes |
| 1 medium onion |
| 2 fat cloves garlic |
| a bunch of fresh parsley and basil |
| olive oil |
| 2tbs grated parmesan cheese |

# STUFFED COURGETTES

**PROTEIN**

Heat the oven to 180°C/350°F/gas 4. Boil the courgettes for 7–8 minutes. Halve them, scoop out the centres and put the shells in a flat, ovenproof dish. Fry the chopped onion and garlic in the oil, then add the celery, chopped tomatoes, parsley, and chopped courgette flesh. Simmer for 5 minutes, uncovered. Season. Pile into the shells, and cover with grated cheese. Bake for 20–25 minutes.

| INGREDIENTS |
| --- |
| 4 large courgettes |
| 1 large onion, finely chopped |
| 1 clove garlic |
| 2tbs olive oil |
| 2 celery sticks, chopped |
| 400g/14oz can of tomatoes |
| 2tbs fresh parsley, chopped |
| salt and pepper |
| 125g/4oz grated cheese |

# GRATIN OF CAULIFLOWER AND BROCCOLI★

### INGREDIENTS

| |
|---|
| 500g/1lb broccoli |
| 500g/1lb cauliflower florets |
| 2 egg yolks |
| 300ml/½pt milk |
| 175g/6oz low-fat soft cheese |
| 2tsp mustard seeds |
| salt and pepper |
| 50g/2oz peeled walnuts |
| 50g/2oz grated emmenthal cheese |

Steam the broccoli and cauliflower for 5–8 minutes. Beat the egg yolks into the milk, and bring slowly to the boil, stirring all the time. Remove from the heat. Add the soft cheese, mustard seeds, seasoning to taste, and half the walnuts.

Heat the grill. Arrange the cauliflower and broccoli in an ovenproof dish, alternating the colours, and pour over the sauce.

Sprinkle the rest of the walnuts and the grated cheese on top, and put under hot grill until a golden, bubbling crust has formed on top.

PROTEIN

# MARINATED RED CABBAGE WITH MUSTARD

### INGREDIENTS

| |
|---|
| 450ml/¾pt red wine |
| 2 cloves |
| 2 bay leaves |
| 6 juniper berries |
| 3 cloves garlic, peeled and halved |
| 1tsp honey |
| 1tsp lemon juice |
| 1 small red cabbage |
| 2–3tbs olive oil |
| 1tsp strong mustard |
| salt and pepper |

Put the wine in a pan with the cloves, bay leaves, juniper berries, garlic cloves, honey, and lemon juice. Bring to the boil and simmer for 20 minutes.

Trim off the outer leaves of the cabbage, quarter it, trim away the thick stalk and the heavier ribs, and slice finely. Put the sliced cabbage in a bowl, pour over the hot marinade, and leave in a cool place for at least 24 hours.

When you are ready to serve the dish, take the red cabbage out of its marinade, and arrange it in a plain white dish. Stir the mustard and a little pepper and salt into the olive oil. Pour the dressing over the cabbage.

PROTEIN

# AUBERGINES STUFFED WITH CHEESE★

**PROTEIN**

*This filling and delicious dish comes from Arto der Haroutunian's* Classic Vegetable Cookery.

Heat the oven to 180°C/350°F/gas 4. Remove the stalks and cook the aubergines in boiling water for about 5 minutes, or until just tender – check by piercing with a knife. Drain. When cool, halve lengthways and scoop out most of the flesh – be careful not to damage the skins. Chop up the flesh, and put it in a bowl. Add the butter, onion, cheese, eggs, parsley, paprika, and black pepper. Check before you add salt – some cheeses are saltier than others. Mix well.

Arrange the aubergine shells in a shallow, greased, ovenproof dish. Spoon the mixture into the shells. Don't fill them too full – any surplus can be cooked in between the shells. Bake in the oven for about 45 minutes, until golden and bubbly.

| INGREDIENTS |
| --- |
| 4 medium aubergines |
| 25g/1oz melted butter |
| 1 medium onion, finely chopped |
| 175g/6oz feta cheese, or edam or cheddar, grated |
| 2 small eggs, beaten |
| 2tbs fresh parsley, finely chopped |
| a good pinch of paprika |
| freshly ground black pepper and salt, to taste |

# FENNEL WITH MOZZARELLA★

**PROTEIN**

Heat the oven to 200°C/400°F/gas 6. Clean the fennel, reserving some of the feathery green tops for garnishing. Slice the bulbs, and cook in boiling, lightly salted water until just *al dente*. Drain them and blot dry. Melt the butter in a pan, and turn the slices of fennel gently in it until they start to take on a little colour. Arrange the fennel in an oiled casserole. Slice the mozzarella cheese thinly, and arrange on top of the fennel. Beat the eggs and cream together with the parmesan cheese and parsley, and pour over the mozzarella and fennel layers. (If you use grated cheddar cheese, sprinkle it on top.) Bake until the top is golden and bubbling – about 20 minutes.

| INGREDIENTS |
| --- |
| 4 fine heads of fennel |
| 2tbs melted butter |
| salt and pepper |
| 200g/7oz mozzarella or grated cheddar cheese |
| 4 eggs |
| 150ml/¼pt single cream |
| 1tbs grated parmesan cheese |
| 2tbs fresh chopped parsley |

# GREEN BEAN STEW

### INGREDIENTS

| |
|---|
| 500g/1lb green beans |
| 5–6tbs olive oil |
| 1 onion, finely sliced |
| 3 cloves garlic, chopped |
| 500g/1lb ripe tomatoes, or a 400g/14oz can |
| water |
| 1tbs lemon juice |
| salt and pepper |

Wash, top and tail, and halve the beans. Heat the oil in a heavy pan, and fry the onion and garlic for a minute or so – don't let them take on colour. Add the beans and fry for another minute or so. If you use fresh tomatoes, skin and chop them. Add these – or the canned tomatoes – together with just enough water to cover the beans. Add the lemon juice. Bring to the boil, and simmer until the beans are done, 10–15 minutes. Season to taste.

PROTEIN

# BRUSSELS SPROUTS GRATIN

### INGREDIENTS

| |
|---|
| 500g/1lb small Brussels sprouts |
| 50g/2oz butter |
| 2tbs grated cheddar cheese |
| salt and pepper |

Preheat the oven to 200°C/400°F/gas 6. Trim the sprouts and wash in plenty of running water. Drain them and cook in lightly salted, boiling water for about 10–15 minutes – they should be just *al dente* – still firm when you stick a knife-point into them. Drain. Put the butter in an ovenproof casserole and heat. When the butter has melted, add the sprouts and roll them around until they are well coated. Sprinkle the cheese over the sprouts, season, and put in the oven for about 10 minutes – long enough for the cheese to turn bubbly and golden.

PROTEIN

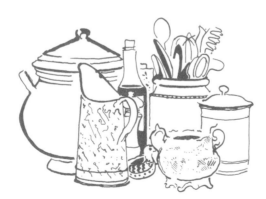

# GREEN BEANS PARMIGIANO

**PROTEIN**

Top and tail the beans, and remove the strings if necessary. Put in a pan of boiling water, and simmer until tender. Drain (reserve the water for stock), and keep hot. Melt the butter and heat the oil in the same pan, add the garlic, and fry for a minute – *no longer*. Add the beans, toss, and reheat gently for 3–4 minutes. Add the parmesan, stir through, and serve sprinkled with the parsley.

| INGREDIENTS |
| --- |
| 500g/1lb French beans |
| 50g/2oz butter |
| 1tbs olive oil |
| 1 large clove garlic, finely chopped |
| salt and pepper |
| 1tbs grated parmesan cheese |
| 1tbs fresh parsley, chopped |

# FULL OF BEANS

**PROTEIN**

Drain the beans, put in separate pans, and cover with plenty of cold water. Bring to the boil and boil rapidly for 10 minutes, then turn the heat down, cover, and simmer for about an hour, or until the beans are tender. Drain, reserving the liquid.

Heat the oil in a heavy pan, add the onion and garlic, and let them soften. Add the carrots, courgettes, celery, tomatoes, thyme, and seasoning to taste. Add enough of the bean cooking water to moisten. Cover and simmer for about 15 minutes, adding more of the bean water if necessary, until all the vegetables are soft. Add the beans and more liquid as needed. Cover, heat through gently, and serve.

| INGREDIENTS |
| --- |
| 50g/2oz dried butter beans, soaked overnight |
| 50g/2oz dried red kidney beans, soaked overnight |
| 1tbs olive oil |
| 1 large onion, finely chopped |
| 2 cloves garlic, finely chopped |
| 2 large carrots, sliced |
| 2 courgettes, sliced |
| 2 celery sticks, sliced |
| 200g/7oz can tomatoes |
| a small sprig of fresh thyme, or a pinch of dried thyme |
| salt and pepper |

# VEGETABLE DISHES FOR PROTEIN OR STARCH MEALS

## GREEN BEANS WITH GARLIC AND CHILLI

### INGREDIENTS

| |
| --- |
| 500g/1lb green beans |
| 1tbs olive oil |
| 2 cloves garlic, peeled and finely chopped |
| 1 dried red chilli pod, seeds removed |

*Chillies can vary in the intensity of their fieriness and if you don't eat them often, you may prefer to use just a couple of fragments of the papery skin. Even this suggestion of chilli will give an agreeable bite to your beans.*

Wash, then top and tail the beans. Cook them until just tender in boiling water. Drain, but reserve the water for stock. Heat the oil in a heavy pan, add the garlic and chilli, and let them sizzle for a few seconds. Add the beans, toss together thoroughly, and serve.

NEUTRAL

## PEAS WITH LETTUCE

### INGREDIENTS

| |
| --- |
| 3 or 4 small, or 2 large, lettuces – the round, floppy kind is best |
| 75g/3oz butter |
| 1.5kg/3lbs of young peas in their pods, shelled |
| 4–5 fat spring onions |
| 2–3 leaves of mint |
| 1tbs chopped fresh parsley |
| 1 teacup light vegetable stock |
| salt and pepper |

*This is good for when you have a glut of lettuce – and so delicious it could be the basis of a light meal. For a Starch meal, serve* crudités *of fresh, raw vegetables on the side, and a helping of plain rice, a baked potato, some tiny new potatoes, or a wholewheat roll. For a Protein meal, add some stalks of celery, a piece of your favourite cheese, and fresh fruit.*

NEUTRAL

Peel off the limp or discoloured outer leaves of the lettuce, wash them meticulously under cold running water, drain, and quarter each head. Melt the butter in a casserole, and turn down the heat to low. Add the peas, the onions, cleaned and cut into rings, and the lettuces. Pour over the hot stock, season lightly to taste, cover, and cook at a bare simmer for 25–30 minutes.

Check that there isn't too much liquid after 15 minutes. If there is, remove the cover, and turn up the heat a little to reduce it. Add the chopped mint and parsley. Stir in another nut of butter, and serve.

# VEGETABLE PURÉES

Potatoes are what people often miss most when they first start eating the Hay way: something bland and filling for a protein meal, something to mop up the gravy or sauce. The vegetable purées that follow are all neutral – and can fill this gap nicely.

## CAULIFLOWER AND ARTICHOKE CRUSH

NEUTRAL

Trim the stalk and outer leaves off the cauliflower, but save the tender inner leaves. Cut off the florets, leaving most of the thicker stalk. Put a little water in a heavy pan, bring to the boil, and add the cauliflower florets and the inner leaves. Lower the heat and steam-cook, tightly covered, until the florets are just cooked – tender but still with some bite to them. Add the artichoke hearts, heat through, and drain, reserving the cooking water. Purée in a food processor or blender, together with the oil, and enough of the cooking water to make a firm, not too mushy, purée. Season with nutmeg, and a little salt to taste.

| INGREDIENTS |
| --- |
| 1 cauliflower |
| 4-5 artichoke hearts, bought loose from a delicatessen or canned in oil |
| 2tbs olive oil |
| nutmeg |
| salt |

## ✳ CREAMED ONIONS

NEUTRAL

Peel and finely chop the onions. (Rubbing a cut lemon over your cheeks beforehand actually does help to stop the tears.) Put the onions in a pan with just enough water to cover and simmer until tender (about 40 minutes). Process or blend them to a smooth cream. Reserve any surplus liquid for a soup.

Put the onions back in the pan, season to taste, and stir in a big lump of butter and a scant teaspoon of flour. Cook over the lowest possible heat for 10–15 minutes. Before you serve the dish, stir in the cream, and grate over a little nutmeg.

| INGREDIENTS |
| --- |
| 5–6 large onions |
| salt and pepper, to taste |
| a big lump of butter |
| 1tsp flour |
| 2–3tbs single cream |
| nutmeg |

*quite a bit of salt.*
*Very runny.*
*Yummy. We had ? pasta*

# TURNIP AND CARROT PURÉE

**NEUTRAL**

### INGREDIENTS

| |
|---|
| 250g/8oz young carrots |
| 250g/8oz young turnips |
| 25g/1oz butter |
| 2tbs fresh chopped herbs – parsley, chives, mint, and chervil |
| sea salt and freshly ground pepper |

Scrub and thinly slice the carrots. If the turnips are very young and fresh, scrub them before thinly slicing them, otherwise pare them very finely first. Since one vegetable may take longer to cook through than the other, it's best to cook them separately: each in an inch or so of boiling water, in a tightly covered pan. When the vegetables are just tender, drain them, reserving the cooking water for a soup. If you have one, put them through the coarse sieve of a *mouli-légumes*. Otherwise process the vegetables or blend them very briefly – we're not aiming at babyfood consistency. Add a little of the cooking liquid if the mixture becomes too thick.

Heat the butter in a heavy pan, over a fairly low heat. Add both lots of sieved vegetables, and stir thoroughly. Heat through, season to taste, and just before serving, stir in the fresh herbs, and another nut of butter.

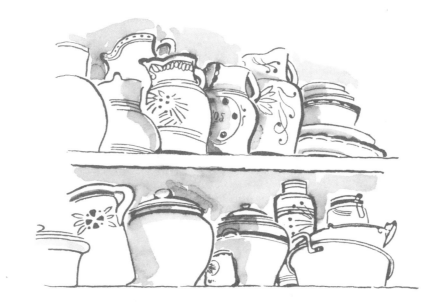

# VEGETABLE DISHES FOR A STARCH MEAL

## SESAME ROAST POTATOES

**STARCH**

Heat the oven to 200°C/400°F/gas 6. The potatoes should be all of a similar size, and not too big. Peel them, and put them in a pan of boiling water. Cook for about 15 minutes. Take the potatoes out and drain them, and let them cool a little – to save your fingers from scalding. Roll them in the sesame seeds. Heat the oil in a baking tin, put in the potatoes, and turn them around until they are well oiled. Leave them to roast for about an hour, or until they are a beautiful golden-brown.

Serve the potatoes with one of the vegetable purées (pp.114–5).

| INGREDIENTS |
| --- |
| 1kg/2lbs potatoes |
| 50g/2oz sesame seeds |
| 2tbs olive oil |

## PUREE OF POTATOES AND CELERIAC

**STARCH**

Have ready a pan containing 1 litre/1³/₄ pints of boiling water, into which you have put the white wine vinegar or the lemon juice. (This will prevent the celeriac from discolouring before it cooks.) Slice the celeriac root in half, then quickly peel off the nobbly outside bits. Slice it fairly thinly and put the slices in the water. Bring to the boil, then lower the heat to a simmer. After 20 minutes add the peeled potatoes, cut into big chunks. Let the 2 cook together until both are ready: about 35–40 minutes in all. (If you misjudge, keep the cooked vegetable hot in a colander over a pan of boiling water.)

When both vegetables are cooked, drain off the liquid and reserve this. Mash both vegetables together, adding a little of their liquid, the butter, and the cream. Add more liquid if you want the purée to be thinner. Season to taste, and sprinkle with the chopped parsley.

| INGREDIENTS |
| --- |
| 1litre/1¾pt water |
| 1tbs white wine vinegar or lemon juice |
| 1 large celeriac |
| 500g/1lb potatoes |

## POTATOES BAKED WITH ROSEMARY

### INGREDIENTS

| |
|---|
| 500g/1lb potatoes |
| 2tbs olive oil |
| a good pinch of rosemary |
| salt |

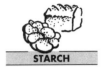

STARCH

*Potatoes baked this way are aromatic and delicious – and not half as high in fat as ordinary roast potatoes.*

Heat the oven to 200°C/400°F/gas 6. Scrub the potatoes, and cut them into cubes the size of giant dice. Put the oil in a baking tin – preferably non-stick – add the potatoes, and roll them around until they are glistening with the oil. Sprinkle them with rosemary, and a little salt. Bake until they are done (about an hour).

## VEGETABLE CURRY

### INGREDIENTS

| |
|---|
| 2 medium potatoes |
| 2 large carrots |
| 2 courgettes |
| 1 onion |
| 2 cloves garlic |
| 2tbs oil |
| 1tsp cumin seeds |
| 1 fresh green chilli or 1 dried red one |
| 1tbs fresh curry powder |
| a few cauliflower florets |
| 1tbs fresh or frozen peas |
| a cupful of water |

STARCH

Scrub the potatoes. Boil them until cooked but not too soft. Cool, and cut them into big cubes. Clean and dice the carrots. Clean and slice the courgettes. Finely slice the onion. Chop the garlic.

Heat the oil in a heavy frying-pan, and add the cumin seeds. Let them sizzle briefly. Add the chilli and let it fry for a few seconds, stirring it about. (If you don't like your food too fiery, slice open the green or red chilli, and shake out the little white seeds. Wash your hands very thoroughly afterwards.) Add the onions and garlic, and let them fry very gently until they are translucent. Stir in the curry powder and sauté for a few minutes.

Add the vegetables, and pour in a cupful of water. Bring to the boil, stir around gently, then cover the pan, and lower the heat. Let the vegetables cook gently together until they are tender. Remove the chilli before serving.

A cucumber salad is pleasantly cooling, served on the side.

# POTATO AND MUSHROOM CASSEROLE

**STARCH**

Heat the oven to 180°C/350°F/gas 4. Wash, peel, and slice the potatoes thinly. Wipe and finely slice the mushrooms. Use half the butter to grease a fairly shallow, ovenproof casserole. Arrange the potatoes and mushrooms in alternating layers, finishing with a layer of potatoes. Lightly season each layer and scatter over it a little of the garlic. Dot the rest of the butter over the top, cover with foil, and bake in the oven for about 1¼ hours.

When the casserole has been cooking for about an hour, remove the foil so that the top browns a little, and push a sharp knife into a potato slice to see how the cooking is progressing. Leave for a further 15 minutes to finish cooking, if necessary.

| INGREDIENTS |
| --- |
| 500g/1lb potatoes |
| 250g/8oz mushrooms |
| 50g/2oz butter |
| 2 cloves garlic, finely chopped |
| sea salt |
| freshly ground black pepper |
| 150ml/¼pt half water and half single cream |

# POTATO GALETTE

**STARCH**

Grate the potatoes into a bowl. Add the spring onions – leave some of the green tops on when you chop them – the parsley, the chives, the well-beaten yolks, and salt and pepper to taste. Mix thoroughly. Heat the oil in a heavy, medium-sized frying-pan. Add the potato mixture and flatten it into a rounded galette shape, then fry very gently until golden-brown underneath. Invert it (with the help of a plate, if necessary), and fry on the other side.

Serve with Fresh Tomato Sauce (p.95) and a tossed green salad.

| INGREDIENTS |
| --- |
| 500g/1lb potatoes, well washed |
| 4–5 spring onions, trimmed and finely chopped |
| 1tbs chopped fresh parsley |
| 1tbs chopped fresh chives |
| 2 egg yolks |
| salt and pepper |
| 2tbs olive oil |

## MUSHROOMS PROVENÇALE

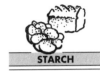

### INGREDIENTS

| |
|---|
| 500g/1lb mushrooms |
| plenty of olive oil |
| salt and pepper |
| 4tbs fresh parsley, finely chopped |
| 3 cloves garlic, finely chopped |
| 4tbs breadcrumbs |

*Big supermarkets offer a variety of mushrooms these days, including the lovely, firm, brown "chestnut" kind, but even the most ordinary of cultivated mushrooms taste delicious in this classic French dish. This is Elizabeth David's recipe, borrowed with a thank you.*

It's difficult to give exact quantities of oil, as some types of mushroom absorb more than others. The mushrooms should not swim in the oil when you sauté them – but don't be too mean either.

Clean and slice the mushrooms, and pour a little oil (1–2tbs) over them, also adding salt and pepper. Leave them to marinate for an hour or so. (This will prevent them from sticking to the bottom of the pan.) Then drain them, and sauté in fresh oil in a small, heavy pan. After 5 minutes' gentle cooking, add the parsley, garlic, and breadcrumbs. When these have absorbed any surplus oil in the pan, the mushrooms are ready to serve.

## KEKI'S ROOT VEGETABLE CASSEROLE

### INGREDIENTS

| |
|---|
| 2 onions |
| 2–3 carrots |
| 1 parsnip |
| 1 large potato |
| 1 raw beetroot, peeled |
| 1 turnip |
| 100–150g/4–6oz broad beans, fresh or frozen |
| 2–3 sprigs of parsley, chopped |
| 1 stick of celery or a small fennel bulb |
| vegetable bouillon powder |

Heat the oven to 190°C/375°F/gas 5. Chop the onions, carrots, parsnip, potato, beetroot and turnip into chunks, and put them in a casserole. Add the broad beans, parsley, and finely sliced celery or fennel. Add just enough water to cover, season with a teaspoonful or so of vegetable bouillon powder, cover the casserole, and cook for about 45 minutes, or until the vegetables are cooked through.

Check from time to time that the dish is not drying out – there should be a little vegetable sauce when it is all done. Serve with a green salad and a wholewheat *chapati*.

# SALADS

A good salad is only as good as the ingredients used in it. The leaves must be as fresh as possible – not stored in the salad compartment since last Saturday's mega-shopping trip. The oil should be of the finest quality you can afford: our own preference is extra-virgin olive oil – store it out of the light. If you use vinegar (we prefer lemon juice), use a good-quality white wine, apple cider, or balsamic vinegar rather than the sharp malt vinegars that ruin so many restaurant salads. The pepper should be freshly ground; the salt, a good sea salt.

Superfoods Salads are garnished with a good sprinkling of fresh green herbs – particularly parsley, mint, and chives. Do consider including wonderful, peppery rocket, basil – especially for tomato salads – the leaves and flowers of nasturtium, and the feathery tops of fennel. Whenever you can, grow your own fresh herbs – on a windowsill if necessary – to ensure a regular supply. Another valuable gadget, we think, is one of those herb-chopping sets consisting of a curved, shallow wooden bowl and crescent-shaped, two-handed blade.

# SALADS FOR PROTEIN MEALS

## MUSHROOM SALAD

**PROTEIN**

*Supermarkets often sell a variety of mushrooms these days. This simple salad is an excellent way to sample their various flavours. The oil needs to be a good one.*

Trim off the stalks, wash the mushrooms carefully, dry them thoroughly, and slice thinly. Arrange in a dish, and season with salt and pepper, oil, and lemon juice. Leave for an hour or so to absorb the flavours. Just before serving, drizzle a little more oil on the mushrooms, and sprinkle with the parsley.

### INGREDIENTS
250g/8oz mushrooms

sea salt

freshly ground pepper

2tbs extra-virgin olive oil

juice of ½ a lemon

1tbs finely chopped parsley

# TOSSED GREEN SALAD

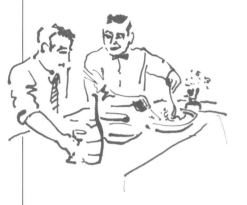

**PROTEIN**

The classic tossed green salad provides a wonderful way to feast on the green leaves that are so important for a healthy diet. Choose as wide a range as possible – different kinds of lettuce including red radicchio, lambs lettuce, oak leaves, cos, iceberg, and butterhead, young spinach or beet greens, and tender young dandelion leaves. They should be thoroughly – and rapidly – washed in cold, salted water, and thoroughly dried: there's nothing worse than a watery salad. Salad-spinners do the job effortlessly for you and seem to us almost as essential a kitchen gadget as a sharp knife. Put the well-dried leaves in a large bowl, torn – not cut – into manageable pieces.

At this point there are two schools of thought. One school maintains that the oil should be added first, and the leaves tossed gently several times until filmed with the oil. Only then should the lemon juice or vinegar, and the other ingredients such as salt, pepper, chopped garlic, and so on, be added. The other school mixes up the dressing and adds it all in one go. If you're pushed for time, it's certainly easier to keep a quantity of dressing ready-made in the refrigerator. The choice is yours.

# MEDITERRANEAN CARROT SALAD

### INGREDIENTS

| |
|---|
| **juice and grated rind of 1 orange** |
| **juice and grated rind of 1 lemon** |
| **2tbs olive oil** |
| **freshly ground pepper** |
| **salt** |
| **500g/1lb carrots** |
| **1tbs pine nuts** |
| **1tbs raisins** |

**PROTEIN**

Scrub the orange and lemon carefully before grating their rinds into a small bowl. Add their juices and the oil, then season with a little pepper and salt. Mix well. Peel and grate the carrots. Put them in a white china dish, then add the dressing, the pine nuts, and the raisins. Toss well, and leave in a cool place for an hour or more.

# RAW ARTICHOKE SALAD

**PROTEIN**

*In Italy, ready-cleaned and pared baby artichokes, floating in bowls of acidulated water, can be bought during the winter months at any street market. But the need to clean them yourself should not deter you from preparing this exquisite, crunchy treat.*

Pick artichokes that are quite small but well-rounded and firm. Have ready a bowl of cold water to which you have added plenty of lemon juice. Trim off the stalks and all but the most tender inner leaves. With a very sharp knife, trim off the tips of these leaves. As each artichoke is ready, drop it into the water.

When you are ready to make the salad, dry the artichokes one at a time. Cut each one in half, remove the chokes, slice very thinly, and put in a white china dish. Mix 2tbs of the lemon juice with the olive oil, season, add to the artichokes, and toss.

If you can get a really good, fresh parmesan cheese, paper-thin slivers are a classic addition to this salad.

| INGREDIENTS |
|---|
| **8 baby globe artichokes** |
| **juice of 2 lemons** |
| **4tbs extra-virgin olive oil** |
| **sea salt** |
| **freshly ground black pepper** |
| **slivers of fresh parmesan cheese (optional)** |

# AVOCADO, SPINACH, AND MUSHROOM SALAD

**PROTEIN**

Wash the spinach thoroughly in several changes of water, dry thoroughly (in a salad-spinner if you have one), and arrange in a deep bowl. Clean the mushrooms, and slice into thin slices. Peel and slice the avocado. Arrange the mushrooms and avocado on top of the spinach, and sprinkle with lemon juice.

At this stage the salad bowl can be covered with a damp cloth, or clingfilm, and put in the refrigerator for not more than half an hour. When you are ready to serve the salad, spoon over the oil, and season to taste. Scatter on top the chopped parsley, and the pine nuts if you are including them. Toss gently just before serving.

| INGREDIENTS |
|---|
| **50g/2oz young spinach leaves** |
| **125g/4oz mushrooms** |
| **1 avocado pear** |
| **1tbs lemon juice** |
| **2 cloves garlic** |
| **2tbs olive oil** |
| **salt and pepper** |
| **1tbs fresh parsley, chopped** |
| **1tbs pine nuts (optional)** |

## FRUIT AND COTTAGE CHEESE SALAD

### INGREDIENTS

| |
|---|
| **2 crisp eating apples** |
| **2 celery stalks** |
| **2 pears** |
| **lettuce leaves** |
| **150g/5oz low-fat cottage cheese** |
| **50g/2oz shelled walnuts** |
| **1tbs fresh parsley, chopped** |
| **Sour Cream or Yogurt Dressing (pp.127)** |

Scrub and slice the apples. Clean and slice the celery. Peel and slice the pears. Arrange them in a circle on a bed of lettuce leaves, on an attractive flat dish. Spoon the cottage cheese into the centre, and scatter the walnuts over the cheese and fruit. Pour over the Sour Cream or Yogurt Dressing. Sprinkle with the chopped parsley, cover, and chill for half an hour before serving.

PROTEIN

## FENNEL SALAD

### INGREDIENTS

| |
|---|
| **2 medium or 1 large head of firm fennel** |
| **plenty of extra-virgin olive oil** |
| **1tbs freshly squeezed lemon juice** |
| **sea salt** |
| **freshly ground black pepper** |

Pull off any damaged outer leaves from the fennel, and cut off the feathery tops, reserving the freshest-looking of the green fronds. Wash and dry thoroughly. Slice the fennel and arrange on a flat dish. Dribble over plenty of olive oil and the lemon juice. Leave in a cool place for at least an hour. Just before serving, season with the salt and pepper to taste, and garnish with some of the reserved fennel fronds.

PROTEIN

## AVOCADO, WALNUT, AND WATERCRESS SALAD

### INGREDIENTS

| |
|---|
| **1 bunch watercress** |
| **2 firm, ripe avocado pears** |
| **4 spring onions, cleaned and finely chopped** |
| **50g/2oz shelled walnuts** |
| **2tbs olive oil** |
| **juice of ½ lemon** |
| **salt** |

*This is a good-looking salad, which should be presented on individual plates.*

Wash and dry the watercress, trim off the stalky bits, and divide between 4 plates. Peel and thinly slice the avocados. Divide them between the plates, and scatter with the chopped spring onions and walnuts. Combine the oil, lemon, and salt. Pour this dressing over the salad ingredients. Cover with a damp cloth or clingfilm, and chill for half an hour before serving.

PROTEIN

# WINTER SALAD ✓ 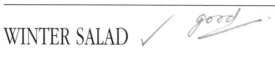 *good*

**PROTEIN**

Soak the apricots overnight, or at least for a couple of hours, in the orange juice.

Clean the cabbage and shred finely, discarding the tough, stalky bits. Mix with the apricots and walnuts. Season.

Make a dressing with the yogurt, honey, and a little grated lemon rind. Toss the salad in the dressing just before serving.

| INGREDIENTS |
| --- |
| 250g/8oz white cabbage |
| 4tbs orange juice |
| 50g/2oz dried apricots |
| 25g/1oz walnuts, chopped |
| salt and pepper |
| 2tbs natural set yogurt |
| 2tsp clear honey |
| grated lemon rind |

# COLESLAW 1

**PROTEIN**

Combine the cabbage, carrots, celery, and apple in a serving bowl. Spoon over the dressing of your choice, toss, cover with clingfilm or a damp cloth, and chill for at least an hour. Just before serving, scatter with the parsley.

| INGREDIENTS |
| --- |
| ½ head green cabbage, cleaned and shredded |
| 2–3 carrots, scrubbed and grated |
| 2–3 celery stalks, cleaned and diced |
| 1 sweet red apple, scrubbed and very finely sliced |
| Sour Cream or Yogurt Dressing (p.127) |
| 1tbs fresh chopped parsley, to garnish |

# RED RADICCHIO, ICEBERG LETTUCE, AND ROCKET SALAD

**PROTEIN**

Pull off the wilted outer leaves of the radicchio, cut off the base, and pull the leaves off separately. If they are too big, tear them (don't cut them) into small pieces. Wash. Trim the iceberg lettuce in the same way, and wash thoroughly. Trim most of the stalks off the rocket, and wash thoroughly. Dry all the leaves together, arrange in a big salad bowl, and dress with the French Dressing.

| INGREDIENTS |
| --- |
| 1 small head red radicchio |
| 1 medium iceberg lettuce |
| plenty of rocket |
| French Dressing I (p.127) |

# GREEK SALAD

### INGREDIENTS

| |
|---|
| 6–8 small tomatoes, washed and quartered |
| 1 small onion, sliced into rings |
| ½ green pepper, cleaned and sliced |
| ½ small cucumber, peeled and sliced |
| 8–10 black olives |
| 125g/4oz feta cheese: if you can't get this, use ricotta or cottage cheese |
| 4–5tbs extra-virgin olive oil |
| dried oregano |
| salt and pepper |

*A meal in itself, this salad needs to be made with the finest possible ingredients: plump black olives, ripe red tomatoes, and extra-virgin olive oil.*

Mix all the ingredients in a plain white china bowl, and toss them gently with the oil. If you use ricotta or cottage cheese – which lacks the firm texture of feta – add it after this stage. Sprinkle with a good pinch of dried oregano, and season with salt and pepper to taste.

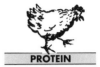

PROTEIN

# FRUIT AND CHEESE SALAD

### INGREDIENTS

| |
|---|
| 2 thick slices of pineapple |
| 2 crisp eating apples – if possible red-skinned |
| juice of 1 lemon |
| 50g/2oz raisins |
| 1 small cucumber, cleaned and diced |
| 2 stalks of celery, chopped |
| 175g/6oz hard cheese, cubed |
| 150g/5oz natural yogurt |
| ½tsp clear honey |
| a pinch of salt |
| 1tbs chopped chives or parsley |
| lettuce leaves |

Cut the pineapple into cubes: if fresh pineapple is not available, use pineapple canned in its own juice. Wash, core, and slice the apples, then toss them in most of the lemon juice – save a little for the dressing. Mix in a bowl the pineapple, apple, washed and dried raisins, cucumber, celery, and cheese. Beat together the yogurt, honey, lemon juice, salt, and fresh herbs, then toss together with the salad. Line individual plates with lettuce leaves, divide the salad into 4 portions, and serve.

PROTEIN

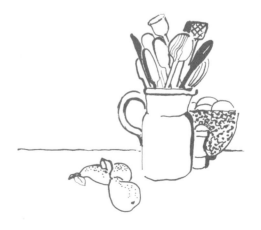

## CABBAGE, CELERY, AND APPLE SALAD

**PROTEIN**

Clean and shred the cabbage. Scrub, core, and thinly slice the apple. Clean and slice the celery. Arrange them all in a dish. Mix together the sour cream, seasoning, lemon juice, and honey, and pour over the salad. If possible, leave to marinate for a couple of hours. Toss, and sprinkle with the parsley just before serving.

| INGREDIENTS |
| --- |
| ½ small white cabbage |
| 1 crisp eating apple |
| 3–4 celery stalks |
| 150g/5oz sour cream |
| 2tbs lemon juice |
| 1tsp clear honey |
| salt and freshly ground pepper |
| 1tbs parsley, freshly chopped |

## AVOCADO, TOMATO, AND MUSHROOM SALAD

**PROTEIN**

*This salad should be dressed at the last minute, so that the fresh taste of each ingredient is preserved.*

Peel and finely slice the avocado. Wash and slice the tomatoes. Clean, trim, and slice the mushrooms. Arrange prettily in a dish, and sprinkle with the lemon juice. (At this point you can cover the dish with clingfilm and keep in a cool place – though preferably not a refrigerator.) Just before serving, sprinkle the olive oil over the salad, season, and garnish with plenty of snipped chives, basil leaves, or finely chopped parsley.

| INGREDIENTS |
| --- |
| 1 ripe avocado |
| 2–3 red tomatoes |
| 150g/5oz mushrooms |
| 1tbs lemon juice |
| 3tbs olive oil |
| salt and freshly ground pepper |
| plenty of fresh chives, basil, or parsley |

## HOT COURGETTE SALAD

**PROTEIN**

Wash and trim the courgettes, then cook them whole in boiling water until just tender: they should still be firm. Drain them, slice quickly, and arrange on a plate, then pour the oil and lemon juice over them. Sprinkle with the parsley and spring onions. Season to taste with salt and freshly ground black pepper.

| INGREDIENTS |
| --- |
| 500g/1lb small courgettes |
| 4tbs olive oil |
| 1–2tbs lemon juice |
| 1tbs fresh parsley, finely chopped |
| 3–4 spring onions, cleaned and finely chopped |
| salt and pepper |

# SALAD DRESSINGS

## FRENCH DRESSING 1

### INGREDIENTS
| |
|---|
| **3tbs extra-virgin olive oil** |
| **1tbs lemon juice** |
| **freshly ground black pepper** |
| **sea salt** |

Combine all the ingredients in a jug and stir vigorously. If making the dressing in a larger quantity, store any that you do not use immediately in a tightly closed bottle or screwtop jar in the refrigerator. Shake the jar well before using the dressing. Optional extras include: plenty of chopped garlic; finely chopped spring onions; a dash of chilli pepper; a teaspoon of Dijon mustard; a pinch of dried herbs.

PROTEIN

## YOGURT DRESSING

### INGREDIENTS
| |
|---|
| **150ml/5oz natural yogurt** |
| **2tbs lemon juice** |
| **2–3 spring onions, cleaned and chopped** |
| **freshly ground pepper** |
| **a touch of sea salt** |

Combine all the ingredients in a blender or food processor. Process until fairly smooth. If using this dressing for a salad containing fruit, omit the salt and pepper, and add a teaspoon of clear honey.

PROTEIN

## SOUR CREAM DRESSING 1

### INGREDIENTS
| |
|---|
| **150ml/5oz sour cream** |
| **2tbs lemon juice** |
| **1tsp clear honey** |
| **a pinch of paprika** |

Beat all the ingredients together, or process in a food processor or blender. If the dressing is to accompany a salad containing fruit, substitute pineapple juice for the lemon juice.

PROTEIN

# SALADS FOR PROTEIN OR STARCH MEALS

## COLESLAW II

**NEUTRAL**

Clean and finely shred the cabbage. Combine with the carrots, celery, spring onions, and raisins. Toss the vegetables in the Sour Cream Dressing. Cover and leave to chill for at least an hour. Just before serving, garnish with the chopped parsley, celery seeds, or caraway seeds.

| INGREDIENTS |
| --- |
| 1½ heads green, white, or red cabbage, or a mixture |
| 1–2 carrots, scrubbed and grated |
| 2–3 stalks of celery, cleaned and diced |
| 2 spring onions, cleaned and finely chopped |
| 1tbs raisins, washed and dried |
| Sour Cream Dressing I or II (p.127 and 132) |
| chopped fresh parsley, or 1tsp celery seeds, or 1tsp caraway seeds |

## BROAD BEAN AND MUSHROOM SALAD

**NEUTRAL**

Put the beans, button mushrooms (cleaned and finely sliced), and the spring onions (trimmed and finely chopped) in a bowl. Wash, dry, and chop the parsley. Pour the olive oil into the bowl, and toss the salad gently – being careful not to break the tender beans. Sprinkle in the lemon juice, finely chopped garlic, salt, and pepper. Sprinkle the parsley over the top.

| INGREDIENTS |
| --- |
| 375g/12oz shelled, young broad beans |
| 125g/4oz button mushrooms |
| 3–4 spring onions |
| a big bunch of fresh parsley |
| 3tbs olive oil |
| 1tsp lemon juice |
| 2 cloves garlic |
| salt and pepper |

## TOMATO SALAD

**INGREDIENTS**

| |
|---|
| **4 tomatoes** |
| **4 cloves garlic** |
| **a good handful of fresh herbs – choose from parsley, chives, mint, or basil, or use all 4, washed, dried, and finely chopped** |
| **freshly ground pepper** |
| **4tbs olive oil** |
| **a little sea salt** |

Wash the tomatoes and slice them finely. Spread the tomatoes in a single layer on an attractive dish. Chop the garlic very finely and sprinkle it over them. Scatter the fresh herbs – the more the better – over the top. Add a little freshly ground pepper. Leave in a cool place while the tomatoes absorb the flavours of the garlic and herbs. Just before serving, add salt to taste, and dribble over the olive oil.

NEUTRAL

## HOT BEETROOT SALAD

**INGREDIENTS**

| |
|---|
| **500g/1lb uncooked beetroots** |
| **1 small onion, finely chopped** |
| **Sour Cream Dressing I or II (p.127 and p132)** |
| **1tbs fresh chopped parsley or chives, or a mixture of both** |

Choose whole beetroots of similar sizes with plenty of stalk. If they are damaged, or cut off too short, their beautiful red juices may drain away into the cooking water. Scrub them gently, and either put them in a big pan of boiling water, and simmer very gently until they are done, or put them in an ovenproof dish in a very low oven for 2–3 hours. They are done when the skin wrinkles easily: DON'T pierce them with a knife to test them. They should be served while they are still hot, if possible.

NEUTRAL

When the beetroots are done, peel off the skins – which will come away easily. Dice them, and arrange in a pretty china bowl. Scatter the spring onions over them, pour over the dressing, and garnish with the chopped fresh herbs.

## CUCUMBER SALAD

**NEUTRAL**

Peel the cucumbers, slice them paper-thin, and put them in a colander with a very little salt, to drain for half an hour or so. Arrange on a bed of shredded lettuce leaves, and garnish with finely chopped spring onions and parsley. Spoon over the dressing of your choice.

| INGREDIENTS |
| --- |
| 1 large or 2 small cucumbers |
| lettuce leaves |
| 4 spring onions, cleaned and very finely chopped |
| 1tbs parsley |
| French or Sour Cream Dressing I or II (p.127 and 132) |

## RED SALAD

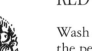

**NEUTRAL**

Wash and slice the tomatoes. Wash, halve, and slice the pepper, removing the small seeds and the woolly inner ribs. Clean and slice the radishes – use the green tops, too, if they are still fresh. Wash and dry the radicchio leaves. Arrange the tomatoes, pepper, and radishes on a bed of shredded lettuce. Drizzle over the dressing, and garnish with the chopped fresh herbs.

If you have a small, uncooked beetroot, peel it, and shred it over the salad at the last moment.

| INGREDIENTS |
| --- |
| 3 tomatoes |
| 1 ripe red pepper |
| 1 bunch of radishes |
| 1 small head of red radicchio |
| Sour Cream Dressing (p.127 and 132) |
| 1tbs fresh chopped parsley, with chives or basil if possible |

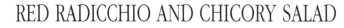

## RED RADICCHIO AND CHICORY SALAD

**NEUTRAL**

Wash the radicchio and tear its leaves into pieces. Clean and slice the chicory. Add the French Dressing and toss the salad thoroughly. Sprinkle lavishly with fresh chopped herbs of your choice.

| INGREDIENTS |
| --- |
| 1 head of red radicchio |
| 2 plump heads of chicory |
| French Dressing I or II (p.127 and 132) |
| fresh chopped herbs |

# CUCUMBER AND WATERCRESS SALAD

| INGREDIENTS |
| --- |
| 1 cucumber |
| salt |
| 1 bunch of watercress |
| 2tbs olive oil |
| 1tbs single cream |
| salt and pepper |

Peel the cucumber and slice into paper-thin slivers. Arrange the slices in a colander, sprinkle with salt, and allow to drain for a few minutes. Wash and trim the watercress. Rinse and dry the cucumber, then combine with the watercress. Combine the olive oil with the cream and seasoning. Dress the salad and serve immediately.

NEUTRAL

# CAULIFLOWER AND CELERY SALAD

| INGREDIENTS |
| --- |
| 1 head of cauliflower |
| 2 celery stalks |
| Sour Cream Dressing I or II (p.127 and 132) |
| fresh parsley |

Wash and dry the cauliflower, then break it up into small florets. Chop the celery and combine with the cauliflower. Pour the dressing over the salad and toss thoroughly. Leave to marinate for at least an hour. Garnish with chopped parsley.

NEUTRAL

# WATERCRESS AND MUSHROOM SALAD

| INGREDIENTS |
| --- |
| 125g/4oz mushrooms |
| Sour Cream Dressing I or II (p.127 and 132) |
| 50g/2oz spinach |
| 1 bunch of watercress |

Clean the mushrooms and slice them finely. Dress the mushrooms with the dressing, and serve on a bed of washed and dried spinach. Garnish with washed and trimmed watercress.

NEUTRAL

# FENNEL AND WATERCRESS SALAD

| INGREDIENTS |
| --- |
| 2 heads of fennel |
| 1 bunch of watercress |
| French Dressing I or II (p.127 and 132) |

Trim and slice the fennel. Clean and trim the watercress. Combine them in a bowl, add the dressing, and toss thoroughly.

NEUTRAL

# SALAD DRESSINGS FOR STARCH MEALS

## FRENCH DRESSING II

**STARCH**

Combine the ingredients in a cup or jar, then stir or shake vigorously.

| INGREDIENTS |
| --- |
| **3tbs olive oil** |
| **1tsp lemon juice** |
| **2–3 spring onions, very finely chopped** |
| **sea salt** |
| **freshly ground black pepper** |

## SOUR CREAM DRESSING II

**STARCH**

Combine all the ingredients, and stir well.

| INGREDIENTS |
| --- |
| **150ml/5oz sour cream** |
| **1tbs tomato juice** |
| **1tsp lemon juice** |
| **a sprinkling of paprika** |

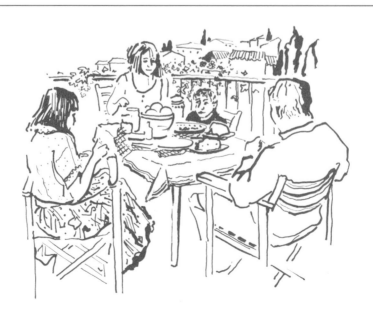

# GRAINS AND PASTA FOR STARCH MEALS

## BARLEY AND MUSHROOM CASSEROLE

| INGREDIENTS |
| --- |
| outer stalks and leaves of a big bunch of celery |
| 1 large onion |
| 1 bunch parsley stalks |
| 900ml/1½pts water |
| 50g/2oz butter |
| 50g/2oz onion, finely chopped |
| 250g/8oz mushrooms, thinly sliced |
| 250g/8oz pot barley |
| ½tsp dried marjoram |
| sea salt and freshly ground pepper |
| fresh parsley, chopped, to garnish |

*This recipe comes from Colin Spencer's inviting collection of Gourmet Vegetarian Dinner Party Menus in Cordon Vert.*

*If you prefer to use nutritionally superior pot barley, cook it beforehand like this: heat 1tsp of oil in a heavy pan, add the well-washed barley, and enough of the celery stock to cover it by a good 5cm/2in. Bring to the boil, cover, and cook over the lowest possible heat or in a moderate oven for about an hour, until the grains are tender. To make the casserole, cook the mushrooms and onions in the butter, until the mushroom juices begin to run. Add the marjoram and the carefully drained barley. Season to taste, and add just enough of the remaining celery stock to moisten the casserole. Heat through over a low heat for a few minutes, then stir in a nut of butter. Sprinkle with parsley and serve.*

Make a stock with the celery, cleaned and chopped; the onion, peeled and cut into chunks; parsley stalks, and water. Bring to the boil and simmer for half an hour, then blend or process, and strain.

Heat the butter in a heavy casserole. Cook the onions and mushrooms for a few minutes, then stir in the barley and cook until the barley begins to absorb the pan juices. Add the marjoram, celery stock, and seasoning, bring to the boil, and simmer for 20 minutes. When the barley is tender, remove the casserole from the heat, turn out into a serving dish, and sprinkle with the parsley.

# MACROBIOTIC MILLET

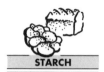

**STARCH**

*This is the way they cook millet at Rome's Centro Macrobiotico Italiano – it's as good as any risotto. If you have never tasted millet before, try this delicious, spicy dish, and add a new grain to your repertoire!*

Toast the millet in a dry pan over a gentle heat for 3–4 minutes. Remove and reserve. Heat the oil in the pan, and melt the onion in it. Add the millet, ground almonds, parsley, chilli, tamari, and water. Bring to the boil, and boil vigorously for 5 minutes. Cover the pan tightly with its lid and cook the millet over a very low heat for 30–40 minutes, or until the water has all disappeared.

| INGREDIENTS |
| --- |
| 250g/8oz millet grains |
| 1 medium onion |
| 1tbs olive oil |
| 1tbs ground almonds |
| 1tbs parsley, very finely chopped |
| 1 small dried chilli |
| 1tbs tamari sauce |
| 450ml/¾pt water |

# PEPPERS STUFFED WITH RICE

**STARCH**

Preheat the oven to 190°C/375°F/gas 5. The cooked rice should still be warm and moist when you stuff the peppers with it, so plan accordingly. First prepare the peppers. Wash them thoroughly, and at the stalk end slice off a lid which you should keep to replace during cooking. It also helps to take a sliver off the other end, so that they don't overbalance during cooking – but take care not to make a hole when you do so. Carefully scoop out the fleshy ribs and all the seeds.

Cook the rice as described on p.136. Slice the onion, heat the oil, and fry the onions until just translucent. Add the pine nuts and currants or raisins and turn them in the hot oil. Add the onion mixture and the fresh herbs to the rice. Season to taste and stuff the peppers. Replace their lids, and put them in a baking tin with boiling water to come about halfway up. Pour 1tbs oil over them, cover with foil, and bake for 30–40 minutes. This dish is delicious served hot or cold.

| INGREDIENTS |
| --- |
| 4 large red, yellow, orange, or green peppers, or 1 of each |
| For the stuffing: |
| 175g/6oz long-grain brown rice |
| 400ml/just under ¾pt water |
| 1 medium onion |
| 1tbs oil |
| 1tbs pine nuts |
| 1tbs currants or raisins |
| 1tbs chopped fresh parsley |
| 1tbs finely chopped mint |
| sea salt |
| freshly ground black pepper |
| 1tbs oil |

# AUBERGINE AND ONION PILAFF

### INGREDIENTS

| |
|---|
| **250g/8oz long-grain brown rice** |
| **1 large aubergine or 2 smallish ones** |
| **sea salt** |
| **3–4tbs olive oil** |
| **1 onion, finely chopped** |
| **1 clove garlic, finely chopped** |
| **freshly ground pepper** |
| **fresh parsley or mint, chopped** |

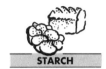
STARCH

Cook the rice as in the recipe on p.136 and keep hot. Cover the casserole, swathe it in several newspapers, and wrap a blanket around it.

Wash the aubergines, remove the stalks, halve them, and cut them into small cubes. Put in a colander, sprinkle with salt, and leave to drain for half an hour. Rinse and dry them thoroughly.

Heat the oil, and fry the onion and garlic until they are just taking on colour. Remove them with a slotted spoon and reserve. Put in the aubergine cubes and fry them. Turn them over several times, until they are taking on colour and well done. Return the onion and garlic to the pan, season, and add a little more oil if necessary. Add the rice. Stir around so that the rice absorbs some of the flavoured oil. Cover, and reheat over a very low flame, or in a very slow oven, for about 10 minutes. Scatter with chopped parsley or mint, or both of these, and serve.

# HENRI'S MUSHROOM RAGOUT WITH RICE

### INGREDIENTS

| |
|---|
| **250g/8oz long-grain brown rice** |
| **900ml/1½pts chicken or vegetable stock** |
| **250g/8oz mushrooms** |
| **1 medium onion** |
| **50g/2oz butter** |
| **1tbs wholewheat flour** |
| **150ml/5fl oz chicken or vegetable stock** |
| **a pinch of nutmeg** |
| **salt and pepper** |

STARCH

The rice can be cooking while you make the ragout. You will need twice its dry volume of stock for cooking, about 600ml/1pt of the stock specified. Wash the rice thoroughly under running water, and put in a heavy pan with the stock. Add a pinch of sea salt, if the stock is not already seasoned. Bring to the boil, cover, lower the heat, and cook until done – about 30–35 minutes.

Meanwhile, wipe the mushrooms clean, then trim and slice them. Slice the onion. Melt the butter in a pan, add the onions and mushrooms, and cook gently for about 5 minutes until they soften, and the mushroom juices start to run. Add the flour and stir it around. Cook for a few minutes without browning. Add the remaining stock – about 300ml/½pt – very hot, and a little at a time, stirring well. Simmer for 15–20 minutes, season, sprinkle with a pinch of nutmeg, and serve with the rice.

# STIR-FRIED VEGETABLES WITH RICE

**STARCH**

*The assortment of vegetables here is just a suggestion. Use whatever is available, fresh, and in season. This dish is best cooked in a wok. If you don't have one, use an ordinary frying-pan, and a minimum amount of oil. Turn the vegetables quickly so that they don't soak up too much oil.*

First cook the well-washed rice. Put it in a heavy pan, and add the vegetable stock. Bring to the boil, lower the heat, cover tightly, and cook for 30–40 minutes. Remove the pan from the heat, uncover it, and let the rice dry out while you begin to prepare the vegetables.

Heat the oil, add the onion and carrots, and turn them in the hot oil for a few minutes. Add the butter and the other vegetables, and raise the heat. Turn the vegetables around briskly for 2–3 minutes, then season, add the rice, and mix well. Pour over the hot stock, and the soy sauce or tamari. Lower the heat, cover, and simmer for about 10 minutes.

| INGREDIENTS |
| --- |
| **175g/6oz long-grain brown rice** |
| **400ml/just under ¾pt vegetable stock** |
| **2tbs oil** |
| **1 onion, thinly sliced** |
| **1tbs butter** |
| **2 carrots, peeled and cut into very small cubes** |
| **2 leeks, cleaned and finely sliced** |
| **2 small courgettes, cleaned and finely sliced** |
| **1 stick of celery, cleaned and finely sliced** |
| **a chunk of cabbage, washed and sliced** |
| **250ml/¼pt vegetable broth** |
| **2tbs soy sauce or tamari** |

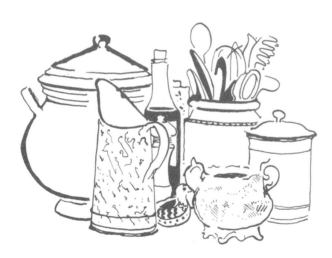

# RAW VEGETABLE RISOTTO

### INGREDIENTS

| |
|---|
| 250g/8oz long-grain brown rice |
| salt |
| 3–4 medium-sized ripe red tomatoes, or 8–10 cherry tomatoes |
| ½ cucumber |
| 4 spring onions |
| 4 young carrots |
| 4 radishes |
| 3 tiny new courgettes |
| 1tbs fresh baby peas |
| 2 cloves garlic |
| 125ml/4fl oz extra-virgin olive oil |
| sea salt and freshly ground black pepper |
| a bunch of chives, chopped small |
| a big bunch of parsley, finely chopped |

*Vegetables used for this fresh, spring or summer dish should be the smallest and freshest of the season.*

STARCH

Wash the rice quickly in a sieve under running water. Cook it in twice its own volume of boiling water, with a little salt added, for about 40 minutes; do this either in a slow oven, or on top of the cooker, over the lowest possible heat, in a tightly sealed pan. Check once or twice to see how it's progressing – but don't stir it. When it is cooked, turn off the oven or remove from the heat, and leave uncovered for about 10 minutes. The rice should be dry and well separated by this time.

Meanwhile, prepare the vegetables. Wash the tomatoes, peel them (just dunk them into boiling water for few minutes so that the skins peel off easily), and chop them very finely. Peel and finely dice the cucumber; clean and chop the spring onions, carrots, radishes, and courgettes, all into the smallest possible pieces. Put them all in a bowl with the peas. Finely chop the garlic, and add it to the bowl, then pour in the olive oil. Season – with great restraint! Leave to marinade in a cool place for a good half hour, so that the oil absorbs some of the fresh, delicate flavours.

While the rice is still tepid, put it in a white china bowl, and pour over the vegetable-flavoured oil sauce. Sprinkle with the green herbs and serve.

# ANGELA'S SPICED CHICKPEA CASSEROLE

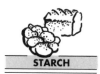

STARCH

*Travel writer Angela Humphery is an inspired and enthusiastic cook, drawing on an eclectic mix of ethnic inspiration for the many delicious dishes she sets before her friends. "This casserole," says Angela, "is a cross-cultural dish, incorporating Middle Eastern chickpeas, Hungarian peppers and paprikas, Greek aubergines, and British spuds."*

Soak the chickpeas in cold water overnight, then put them in a big pan of boiling water. Cook briskly for 10 minutes, then turn the heat down to a simmer. Cook, covered, until soft – anything from 1–2 hours. Drain.

Slice the aubergines, and leave in a colander, sprinkled with a little salt, to drain for half an hour. Rinse and blot dry. Heat the oil and fry the onions, remove them with a slotted spoon, and set aside – first blotting off excess oil with a paper towel. Fry the aubergines in the same oil – you may need to add a little more; remove and blot dry. Do the same with the peppers and tomatoes.

Heat the oven to 190°C/375°F/gas 5. Make layers of each of the vegetables in an ovenproof casserole, together with the chickpeas. Add the garlic, a generous pinch each of the chilli, paprika, and allspice, and season. Mix the olive paste and tomato purée with 2tbs of water and pour it into the casserole dish. Pour in enough water to come almost to the top, cover, put it in the oven, and cook for about 1½ hours. Serve with warm wholemeal *pita* bread and a green salad.

## INGREDIENTS

| |
| --- |
| **250g/8oz dried chickpeas** |
| **2tbs oil** |
| **2 large onions, sliced** |
| **2 large aubergines** |
| **3 peppers – one red, one green, and one yellow, cleaned and sliced** |
| **2 large potatoes** |
| **fresh coriander** |
| **2 cloves garlic** |
| **chilli powder** |
| **paprika** |
| **allspice** |
| **salt and pepper** |
| **2tsp olive paste** |
| **2tsp tomato purée** |

# PASTA

The pasta loved by Italians is usually made from refined flour. However, Italians themselves are eating increasing amounts of *pasta integrale*, or wholewheat pasta, especially in the form of fresh tagliatelle now sold by many bakers. Wholewheat pasta is chewier and tastier than ordinary pasta, it takes rather longer to cook than ordinary white, and it is harder to judge when it's cooked to *al dente* perfection. Wholewheat pasta is well worth experimenting with, and so is buckwheat pasta, which has a distinctive flavour of its own. If, however, you still prefer ordinary pasta made from refined flour, choose one of these simple vegetable sauces to accompany it, make the dish with wonderful extra-virgin olive oil, and eat the pasta with a green salad and a dark green, leafy vegetable on the side, to make up for the missing fibre and essential B vitamins.

Whether wholewheat or ordinary refined, pasta should be cooked in the biggest pan you own, in plenty of water, salted – about a level tablespoon for four people – just before you add the pasta. The water should be boiling vigorously when the pasta goes in – all at once, please, and NEVER broken. If you're cooking short, fat, or more solid types of pasta, add a tablespoon of oil to prevent it from sticking. The pasta is cooked when still JUST chewy or *al dente*: a moment that can come and go with alarming speed. At this point it should come straight off the heat, go into a colander to drain, and then be transferred into a hot dish ready to be dressed with its sauces and served. In other words, sauce, dish, colander, and consumers should all be waiting for the pasta, rather than the other way round.

Depending on appetites, allow about 100–125g or around 4oz of pasta per person. On the whole, the more convoluted the pasta shape, the thicker the sauce needs to be. For the simplest Garlic, Oil, and Herb Sauce, nothing could be nicer than fine *spaghettini*. For the Cauliflower and Broccoli Sauce (p.141), you might choose twists, the little ear-shaped pasta called *orechiette*, or shells.

## GARLIC, OIL, AND HERB SAUCE

| INGREDIENTS |
| --- |
| **3 cloves garlic** |
| **8tbs olive oil** |
| **plenty of fresh chopped herbs – parsley, mint, basil, or chervil** |

Crush the garlic, stir it into the oil together with the chopped herbs, and leave to macerate for at least half an hour. When the pasta is ready, simply pour the sauce over it.

**STARCH**

## TOMATO, GARLIC, AND BASIL SAUCE

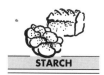

STARCH

Peel the tomatoes, put in a blender and, while it is running, add enough olive oil in a fat trickle to make a thick sauce. Remove from the blender, and add the very finely chopped parsley and basil, the seasoning, and the olives. A few flakes of dried red chilli are an optional extra.

This sauce should be added to the pasta as soon as it is cooked and drained.

| INGREDIENTS |
| --- |
| 500g/1lb ripe tomatoes |
| olive oil |
| 12 cloves garlic |
| a handful of basil leaves |
| a handful of parsley |
| salt and pepper |
| half a dozen black olives, washed, stoned, and halved |
| a few flakes of dried red chilli (optional) |

## RED PEPPER SAUCE

STARCH

Clean and finely slice the onion. Clean the peppers, eliminating the seeds and fleshy ribs. Put both ingredients in a blender or food processor. Add the cream and blend again. Season to taste. Add the sauce to the hot cooked pasta and serve sprinkled with the parsley.

| INGREDIENTS |
| --- |
| 1 medium onion |
| 3 medium red peppers, or 2 red and 1 yellow |
| 150ml/5fl oz single cream |
| salt and pepper |
| a big bunch of parsley, very finely chopped |

## PIQUANT RED SAUCE

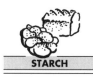

STARCH

Peel the tomatoes, then blend or process them to a thick paste. Peel and finely chop the garlic. Split and deseed the chillies – wash your hands carefully afterwards! Clean and finely chop the parsley and herbs. Wash and very finely chop the celery. Stir all the ingredients together, season, and finally add the olive oil.

| INGREDIENTS |
| --- |
| 750g/1½lbs ripe red tomatoes |
| 2–3 cloves garlic |
| 1 or more dried red chillis, according to taste |
| fresh parsley, basil, and oregano or marjoram |
| 1 stick of celery |
| salt and pepper |
| 2tbs olive oil |

# CAULIFLOWER AND BROCCOLI SAUCE

### INGREDIENTS

**500g/1lb green broccoli florets, or 250g/8oz each cauliflower and green broccoli florets**

**4tbs olive oil**

**1 medium onion**

**1tbs pine nuts**

**1tbs raisins, previously soaked in water for a couple of hours**

**salt and pepper**

Thoroughly wash the cauliflower or broccoli and break into small florets. Slice the onion. Heat the oil in a pan and soften the onion in it. Add the pine nuts and raisins. Cook the cauliflower or broccoli in a panful of lightly salted water (enough to cook the pasta in afterwards), until tender but still chewy. Drain – reserving the water – and add to the raisins, onion, and pine nut mixture. Season to taste. Cook the pasta in the broccoli water.

STARCH

# SICILIAN FENNEL PASTA

### INGREDIENTS

**1 head of fennel**

**4tbs olive oil**

**1 medium onion, finely chopped**

**50g/2oz raisins, soaked for 30 minutes**

**50g/2oz pine nuts**

**salt and pepper**

**500g/1lb pasta of your choice**

*In Sicily they use short, fat tubes of pasta called* rigatoni, *but you can use whatever shape you fancy, including classic fine* spaghettini.

Heat the oven to medium hot, 175°C/350°F/gas 4, and have ready a big, ovenproof dish.

Pick a fine, fat head of fennel, with plenty of fresh green fronds. Clean and trim, chopping and saving the fronds for garnishing. Plunge the whole head into a big pan of boiling water for a few minutes. Lift out the fennel, and reserve all the water. Let the fennel drain, then chop finely.

Heat the oil, add the onion, and fry until transparent. Add the fennel, stir, then add the raisins and pine nuts. Season to taste. Keep hot.

Meanwhile, bring the water in which you cooked the fennel back to the boil, and cook the pasta until just *al dente*. Drain, put in the ovenproof dish, add the sauce, and quickly stir it in. Add a dribble of olive oil, and put in the hot oven for a few moments. Just before serving, scatter the green fennel fronds over the dish.

STARCH

# SNACKS FOR PROTEIN MEALS

## TOMATOES STUFFED WITH COTTAGE CHEESE AND TUNA

PROTEIN

Wash the tomatoes carefully, halve them, and remove most of the pulp, taking care not to pierce the skins. Dust a little salt into them, and reserve. Finely chop the tuna, anchovy, and capers. Mix with the parsley, the reserved tomato pulp, and the cottage cheese. Stuff the tomatoes with this mixture. Sprinkle a little parsley over them.

### INGREDIENTS

4 beefsteak tomatoes

150g/5oz cottage cheese

150g/5oz tuna in oil, drained

1 anchovy fillet

1tsp capers

1 bunch of fresh parsley, finely chopped (reserve a little for garnishing)

## CRUDITÉS WITH A DIP

PROTEIN

*A dish of cleaned and trimmed raw vegetables, served with a savoury dip, can be almost a meal in itself. Serve a selection of the suggested ingredients with one of the following dips.*

Wash and deseed the red and yellow peppers, then cut them into strips. Chop the washed carrots into fingers. Slice the celery into strips. Cut the fennel bulbs into chunks. Slice the cucumber into batons. Separate the cauliflower or broccoli into florets. Wash and trim the radishes, spring onions, and cherry tomatoes (these can be left whole).

### INGREDIENTS

red and yellow sweet peppers

young carrots

celery

fennel

cucumber

cauliflower or broccoli

radishes

spring onions

cherry tomatoes

## EASY MACKEREL DIP

PROTEIN

Use mackerel canned in brine, if possible. Drain the fish, detach any bits of spine, and put in a blender or food processor with the rest of the ingredients. Blend or process until smooth. Chill.

### INGREDIENTS

75g/3oz canned mackerel

75g/3oz ricotta cheese

25g/1oz butter

juice of ½ lemon

1tbs finely chopped spring onion

pepper

# COTTAGE CHEESE AND ONION DIP

### INGREDIENTS

**150g/5oz plain cottage cheese**

**1tbs plain yogurt**

**1tbs lemon juice**

**2 or 3 spring onions, trimmed and finely chopped**

**1tbs fresh parsley, finely chopped**

**salt and freshly ground pepper**

Put all the ingredients in a blender or food processor and blend. Chill. Store in the refrigerator until ready to serve.

**PROTEIN**

# PEPPER AND ONION DIP

### INGREDIENTS

**3 spring onions**

**½ small red pepper**

**½ small green pepper**

**125g/4oz cheddar cheese**

**150g/5oz plain yogurt**

**2tsp tomato purée**

**1tbs Mayonnaise (p.144)**

**½tsp Worcestershire sauce**

**a touch of Tabasco sauce, or chilli pepper**

**salt and pepper**

**1tbs chopped chives or parsley, to garnish**

Clean and finely chop the spring onions, and the red and green peppers. Grate the cheese. Mix with the yogurt, and stir in the tomato purée, mayonnaise, and Worcestershire sauce. Season to taste with salt, pepper, and Tabasco or chilli. Chill. Serve garnished with the chives or parsley.

**PROTEIN**

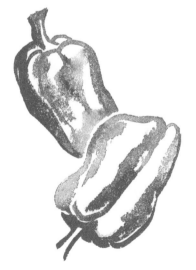

# TUNA AND GARLIC MAYONNAISE★

**PROTEIN**

First make the mayonnaise. Beat the egg yolks into a small bowl, add the garlic and salt, and beat together. Start beating in the oil a drop or so at a time. Once the mayonnaise has begun to thicken, the oil can be added in a steady trickle, then a thin stream. From time to time add a squirt of lemon juice. When all the oil and lemon juice have been added, the mayonnaise should be a wonderful, thick, glossy mixture.

To make the dip, add the tuna, finely chopped spring onions, and parsley to the mayonnaise. Cover with clingfilm, and chill until it is ready to be eaten.

| INGREDIENTS |
| --- |
| **For the Mayonnaise:** |
| **2 egg yolks** |
| **2 cloves garlic, crushed** |
| **a little salt** |
| **200ml/7fl oz extra-virgin olive oil** |
| **1tbs lemon juice** |
| **2tbs tuna tinned in oil (drain off the oil)** |
| **4 spring onions** |
| **2tbs fresh parsley, chopped** |

# COTTAGE CHEESE WITH CUCUMBER AND CHIVES

**PROTEIN**

Turn the cottage cheese into a bowl. Skin, chop, and add the tomatoes. Peel, finely dice, and add the cucumber. Clean and finely chop the spring onions, including some of the green bits, and add to the mixture. Wash and dry the chives, then snip into the mixture. Stir together, season to taste, and serve on a bed of crisp, finely shredded, lettuce.

This mixture can be used to stuff raw red peppers. Pick firm, glossy ones, and clean them thoroughly. Slice enough off the tops to allow you to scoop out the inner seeds and fleshy ribs. Stuff them with the cottage cheese mixture.

| INGREDIENTS |
| --- |
| **300g/10oz cottage cheese** |
| **2 medium-sized red tomatoes** |
| **1 cucumber** |
| **2 spring onions** |
| **1 bunch of chives** |
| **salt and pepper** |
| **lettuce leaves** |

## COURGETTE CROQUETTES

### INGREDIENTS

| |
|---|
| 1tbs olive oil |
| 2 cloves garlic, chopped |
| 1 small onion, sliced |
| 3 or 4 courgettes – about 375g/12oz in weight, cleaned and diced |
| 200g/7oz tomatoes, or a small can |
| salt and pepper |
| 1tbs fresh parsley, chopped |
| 2tbs cheddar cheese, grated |
| 2 egg yolks |
| 4-5tbs wheatgerm |
| oil, for frying |

Heat the oil, and gently fry the garlic and onion for a couple of minutes. Add the courgettes, and cook over a low heat for 15–20 minutes, turning them over quite often. Add the skinned and chopped tomatoes, and cook for another 5–10 minutes, to let some of the moisture evaporate. Let the mixture cool. Season it, then add the parsley, cheese, and beaten egg yolks. Add enough wheatgerm to make the mixture firm, then shape it into croquettes. Dust the croquettes with more wheatgerm, and shallow-fry in hot oil, turning them after 2–3 minutes. Drain on kitchen paper, and serve with a Cucumber and Watercress Salad (p.131) or a plain tossed green salad.

PROTEIN

## TOMATOES STUFFED WITH CELERY, AVOCADO, AND MAYONNAISE★

### INGREDIENTS

| |
|---|
| 4 beefsteak tomatoes |
| 4 celery stalks |
| 4 spring onions |
| 2 avocado pears |
| 4tbs Mayonnaise (p.144) |
| 1tbs lemon juice |
| salt and pepper |
| 2tbs fresh parsley, chopped |

Wash the tomatoes carefully, and halve them. Remove most of the pulp, taking care not to pierce the skins. Dust a little salt into the skins and reserve them. Clean the celery and dice very finely. Clean the spring onions and chop them finely. Peel the avocados, and mash the flesh to a cream, adding the lemon juice. Stir the mayonnaise into the avocado purée. Add the chopped celery, spring onions, the reserved tomato pulp, and most of the parsley – reserve a little for garnishing. Season to taste, and stuff the tomato halves with this mixture. Sprinkle with the reserved chopped parsley.

PROTEIN

# SNACKS FOR A STARCH MEAL

*u, nice* ✳ RICH MUSHROOM PÂTÉ

**STARCH**

Trim and wipe the mushrooms, discarding the stalks. Slice the mushrooms thickly and then cut across into cubes. Chop the onion finely. Warm the cumin and coriander seeds in a frying-pan until they give off a little of their wonderful aroma, then crush them finely (you can put them between 2 layers of baking paper and use a rolling pin if you do not have a pestle and mortar).

Melt the unsalted butter in a pan, add the onion, and cook over a low heat until translucent. Remove with a slotted spoon. Add the mushrooms, and turn up the heat. Fry for about 6 minutes until the mushrooms have shrunk, and given off some of their juice. Add the marsala, then switch off the heat. Return the onions to the pan, add the cumin and coriander, the soya, Worcestershire sauce, and mushroom ketchup. Leave to cool, then put back into the food processor or blender and whizz to a smooth cream. Add the salted butter, a little at a time, whizz again, then scrape out into a pretty china dish that has been lightly oiled. Level the mixture, cover the dish, and chill for several hours. Return to room temperature before serving.

| INGREDIENTS |
| --- |
| 200g/7oz dark field mushrooms or large flat mushrooms |
| 1 small onion |
| ½tsp cumin seeds |
| ½tsp coriander seeds |
| 50g/2oz unsalted butter |
| 1tbs marsala |
| 1 dash soya sauce |
| 1 dash Worcestershire sauce |
| 1tsp mushroom ketchup |
| 50g/2oz salted butter |

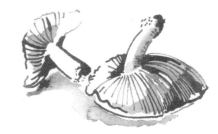

## BLACK OLIVE PÂTÉ

### INGREDIENTS

| |
|---|
| 150g/5oz black olives |
| 1 very small onion |
| 1 clove garlic |
| ½tsp dried thyme |
| 50g/2oz butter |
| salt and pepper, to taste |

STARCH

*These 2 delicious recipes came from Philippa Davenport's* Country Living Country Cook. *Serve the pâtés with fresh, crusty wholemeal baguettes for a picnic or packed lunch, or with hot wholemeal toast as a starter for a Starch meal. For the Black Olive Pâté use only very good olives, packed in olive oil, from a reliable delicatessen. Little squashy Moroccan ones are particularly good.*

Stone the olives, quarter the onion, and finely chop the garlic. Put them all in a food processor with the thyme and process to a paste. Add the slightly softened butter, cut up into dice, a little at a time, and whizz again to create a creamy paste. Check the seasoning, then pack into a small china pot, cover with a piece of foil, and chill for 24 hours.

## ONION QUICHE★

### INGREDIENTS

| |
|---|
| **For the filling:** |
| 50g/2oz butter |
| 1tbs oil |
| 500g/1lb onions |
| sea salt and freshly ground pepper |
| nutmeg |
| 1tbs fresh parsley, chopped |
| 2 egg yolks |
| 125ml/4fl oz single cream |
| **For the pastry:** |
| 125g/4oz plain wholewheat flour |
| a pinch of salt |
| 50g/2oz butter |
| ice-cold water |

STARCH

Heat the butter and oil in a heavy pan. Put in the onions, peeled and sliced as thinly as possible. Cover the pan: the onions should stew rather than fry, over a very low heat, until they are soft and pale gold in colour – allow up to 25 minutes. Stir them occasionally. When they are done, season with salt, pepper, nutmeg, and parsley. Beat together the egg yolks and cream, and add to the onion mixture. Set aside while you make the pastry.

Heat the oven to 200°C/400°/gas 6. Put a baking sheet in the oven to heat. Make the pastry as described in the recipe for Leek Pasties (p.148). Roll it out as thinly as possible and use it to line a very lightly oiled 20cm/8in flan tin. Press the pastry into place with your fingertips. Pour in the filling. Put the flan tin on the hot baking sheet in the oven, and bake for about 30 minutes.

# LEEK PASTIES★

**STARCH**

Clean and trim the leeks, and slice the white parts. Scrub the potato and boil it. Clean and slice the onion. Melt the butter in a heavy pan, put in the onion, and let it soften. Remove the onion with a slotted spoon, reserve, put in the leeks, and let them just soften – they should not change colour. Return the onion to the pan, cover, and allow to stew gently for a few minutes, over a very low heat. Remove the leeks and onion, and set aside in a bowl. Add the flour to the juices in the pan. Stir to make a smooth sauce, and add the cream. Stirring constantly, heat the sauce until it has thickened. Add to the leeks and onion. Add the diced potato. Stir in the parsley, and season to taste. Cool.

Preheat the oven to 200°C/400°F/gas 6. While the filling is cooling, make the pastry. Put the flour in a bowl and mix in a good pinch of salt. Then rub in the butter – the softer this is, the better – until the mixture is the consistency of fine breadcrumbs. Add just enough water to make the dough moist: it should come away easily from the board. On a floured work-surface, knead the dough gently into a rough circle. Roll it out until it is wide enough for you to cut 4 circles, 15cm/6in in diameter, from it. (If you find 100 per cent wholewheat flour too heavy, you can either sieve out the bran, or else buy 85 per cent extraction flour.)

Divide the filling mixture into 4 parts, and put each one on one side of the pastry circle. Brush a little beaten egg yolk around the edges, fold over the other half of the circle, and pinch together, scalloping the edges with a fork. Make a little hole in the top of the pasty, and brush the top with the beaten egg. Place the pasties on a baking sheet, and bake until nicely gilded (approximately 25 minutes).

| INGREDIENTS |
| --- |
| **For the filling:** |
| **4 leeks** |
| **1 medium potato, scrubbed, boiled, and diced** |
| **1 medium onion** |
| **25g/1oz butter** |
| **1tsp flour** |
| **2tbs double cream** |
| **1tbs chopped parsley** |
| **salt and pepper** |
| **1 egg yolk** |
| **For the pastry:** |
| **250g/8oz wholewheat flour** |
| **a little salt** |
| **125g/4oz butter** |
| **ice-cold water** |

## MILLET CROQUETTES

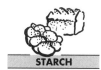

**STARCH**

| INGREDIENTS |
| --- |
| Macrobiotic Millet (p.134), left to cool |
| 1 medium onion |
| 1 tbs oil |
| 2 egg yolks |
| 2 tbs wholewheat flour |
| a little salt and pepper |
| a dash of chilli pepper (optional) |
| oil, for frying |

If you have cooked Macrobiotic Millet and have some left over, this is a good way to use it up. Alternatively, you can cook the millet in just the same way as for Macrobiotic Millet, leaving out the onion and ground almonds, then cool the mixture and use.

Peel and finely slice the onion. Heat the oil, melt the onion, and fry over a gentle heat until soft and golden. Add it to the cold millet mixture, and mix well. Beat the yolk of one of the eggs, and use it to bind the mixture. Shape into croquettes. Season the flour with salt, pepper, and a dash of chilli pepper. Dip each croquette into the beaten yolk of the other egg, roll in the seasoned flour, and fry until golden.

## STUFFED PITA POCKETS

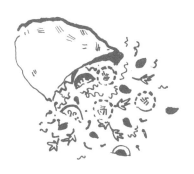

**STARCH**

*Pita* is the everyday bread of the Middle East, round, flat, and only slightly leavened, with a useful hollow middle. Long before the Earl of Sandwich invented the snack that has immortalized his name, *pita* bread was being stuffed with all sorts of delicious goodies to make it a useful portable food. Most supermarkets and delicatessens sell wholewheat *pita* bread.

As a snack there are dozens of delicious possible fillings. For a fresh Middle-Eastern flavour, stuff your *pitas* with fresh tomatoes, stoned and halved, black olives, cucumber slices, sliced radishes – include the tops if these are still green and fresh – spring onions, and a couple of crisp lettuce leaves. Slices of crisp celery and sprigs of watercress are good additions. Season each *pita* with just a touch of dried oregano, and moisten it with a teaspoonful or so of olive oil. Butter and *pita* do NOT go together.

You can also stuff *pitas* with the Rich Mushroom or Black Olive Pâtés (pp.146–7); any of the salads that go with a Starch meal; or just a spot of olive oil, garlic, and fresh chopped herbs.

# PAN BAGNA

**STARCH**

This is another traditional variation on the sandwich theme, this time from Provence. (The name means, literally, soaked bread – because of the olive oil and tomato juice that moistens the loaf while it waits to be eaten.) Pan Bagna, too, is a perfect portable food, since the longer it waits around to be eaten, the juicier it will become.

The basic ingredients are a good olive oil, garlic, ripe, juicy tomatoes, and plump black olives. The rest can vary according to your taste. You might include slices of cucumber, slivers of green or red peppers, chopped spring onions, mashed yolk of hard-boiled eggs, young raw broad beans, and chopped fresh parsley or basil.

The garlic taste is important. Before you stuff the bread, you can simply rub a cut clove over the surface. Alternatively, you can crush a clove of garlic into 1 tbs of olive oil, and allow to marinate for half an hour or so before you use the oil, throwing away the garlic. And, of course, you can use just plain chopped garlic.

Wholewheat baguettes are perfect for Pan Bagna, but you can use wholewheat baps, or indeed almost any kind of roll. Simply slice them in half, fill them with the ingredients of your choice, and moisten with a little olive oil. Press together, with a heavy weight on top, for half an hour.

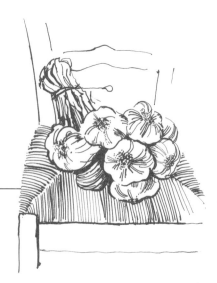

# GARLIC BREAD

| INGREDIENTS |
| --- |
| wholewheat baguettes |
| olive oil |
| garlic cloves, chopped |
| *herbes de provence* |

*Traditionally, garlic bread drips with butter. Try making it with a good, fruity, extra-virgin olive oil instead.*

Slice the baguettes vertically, from one end to the other, but not quite through, so that the slices are still all joined together along the bottom. Have ready a little sauce of olive oil, with very finely chopped garlic and a good sprinkling of *herbes de provence*. Get this ready a good hour ahead, if possible, so that the oil has time to soak up the beautiful aromas of the herbs. Paint the slices liberally on one side with the oil-and-herb mixture. Press the baguette together, wrap in foil, and put in a hot oven for 10–15 minutes.

STARCH

# MUESLI

| INGREDIENTS |
| --- |
| Per person: |
| 1–2tbs oat flakes or oatmeal, or other wholegrain cereal |
| a few raisins |
| a few almonds or other nuts, broken up |
| 3tbs water |
| 1tbs single cream or milk |
| a ripe sweet pear or a banana |

*Muesli is normally thought of as a breakfast dish. When Bircher-Benner first discovered a Swiss shepherd eating his version of it – whole wheat soaked in rich, creamy milk, honey, a few nuts, and an apple – it was the shepherd's supper. If you want a simple, satisfying Starch supper, what could be better?*

Make the muesli a few hours ahead. Put the raisins and the oats or cereal of your choice in a bowl, add the water, and leave in a cool place. When you're ready to eat the muesli, add the nuts, grate in a ripe sweet pear, or slice in a banana. Finally top with cream or milk.

STARCH

# PUDDINGS FOR PROTEIN MEALS

## ORANGE SOUFFLÉ OMELETTE

PROTEIN

*The quantity below serves 2 people – ideally eating cosily in the kitchen, and ready to fall to the moment the omelette is done. We wouldn't advise attempting it for more than 2 – and certainly not for a dinner party.*

Separate the egg yolks from the whites. Beat the yolks in a small bowl, then stir in the orange juice and grated rind, and the sugar. Whisk the egg whites until they stand in peaks, then carefully fold in the yolk mixture. Heat the grill. Melt the butter in a pan. When it is hot, make the omelette in the usual way. When it starts to bubble, slide the pan under the grill and let the omelette puff up and turn golden-brown on top. Serve at once.

| INGREDIENTS |
| --- |
| **4 eggs** |
| **juice and grated rind of 1 orange** |
| **2tsp brown sugar** |
| **a nut of unsalted butter** |

## BAKED APPLES WITH BLACKBERRIES

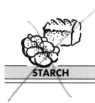

STARCH

*Apples and blackberries have a wonderful autumnal affinity with each other, celebrated in the pies and tarts of childhood memories. Here is a leaner, simpler version of the same partnership.*

Heat the oven to 200°C/400°F/gas 6. Wash the apples, core them, making nice wide holes, and stand them in a greased baking tin. Butter the tops lightly, and stuff the middles with all the blackberries you can cram in. Trickle honey on top of each filling.

Bake for 20–25 minutes, or until the apple skins are glistening and ready to burst. Serve the apples either hot or cold, on their own or with yogurt.

| INGREDIENTS |
| --- |
| **4 large eating apples or Bramleys** |
| **25g/1oz unsalted butter** |
| **250g/8oz blackberries** |
| **2–3tbs clear honey** |

## SPICED APRICOTS

### INGREDIENTS

| |
|---|
| 250g/8oz dried apricots |
| 400ml/¾pt apple juice, white wine, or a fruit herbal tea |
| 1 small stick of cinnamon |
| ½tsp ground nutmeg |
| 4 cloves |
| ½tsp allspice |
| peel of 1 well-scrubbed orange |
| 1tbs honey |

Wash the apricots thoroughly. Put them in a pan with the apple juice, wine or herbal tea, the spices, orange peel, and honey. Bring to the boil. Turn down the heat, and simmer over a very low heat until the apricots are tender. Fresh apricots can be cooked in the same way.

PROTEIN

## RAW APPLE, LEMON, AND HONEY WHIP

### INGREDIENTS

| |
|---|
| juice of 1 lemon |
| 4 crisp eating apples |
| 2tbs clear honey |

Pour the lemon juice into a blender or food processor. Finely peel the apples, core them, cut them into slices, and drop them immediately into the blender or food processor – process immediately. The lemon juice will prevent the apples from turning brown. Add honey to taste, and put in a bowl. Cover with clingfilm, and refrigerate until you're ready to eat the dish – which should be as soon as possible.

PROTEIN

## GOOSEBERRY AND ELDERFLOWER FOOL★

### INGREDIENTS

| |
|---|
| 500g/1lb fresh gooseberries |
| a very little water |
| 1tbs clear honey |
| 150ml/5oz Greek yogurt |

*In her* Fruit Book, *Jane Grigson suggests adding a head or so of fresh elderflowers to the gooseberries while they cook (the seasons just overlap), for their delicate muscat flavour. Be sure to shake them free of wildlife and wash them well.*

Wash, top, and tail the gooseberries. Put them in a pan with no more than 1tbs or so of water, and cook over low heat until the gooseberries disintegrate. Leave to cool. When cold, stir in the honey, and whip in the Greek yogurt.

PROTEIN

# GOOSEBERRY AND APPLE MOUSSE

**PROTEIN**

Put the gooseberries and 1tbs of the apple juice in a pan. Cover and cook over a low flame for a couple of minutes, until the skins have split open. Process and put the purée into a large bowl. Leave to cool. Peel, core, and slice the apples into a pan with 1tbs of apple juice, a sprinkling of cinnamon, and a grating of nutmeg. Cover, and cook until soft. Process and leave to cool. When both purées are cool, drain off any excess juice – use it as a pleasant summer drink, or as an accompaniment to your breakfast yogurt. Stir in the honey, then whisk in the Greek yogurt (save 2tbs for garnishing). Spoon into 4 glasses. Serve chilled, decorated with a swirl of yogurt, and a sprig of apple mint.

For an even fresher summer taste, leave out the cinnamon and nutmeg, and add 2 or 3 more sprigs of mint and a little lemon juice to the apples while they cook.

| INGREDIENTS |
| --- |
| **175g/6oz gooseberries, fresh or frozen** |
| **2tbs apple juice** |
| **2 big crisp eating apples** |
| **2tsp clear honey** |
| **cinnamon** |
| **nutmeg** |
| **150ml/5oz Greek yogurt** |
| **sprigs of apple mint, to decorate** |

# PEACH PUDDING

**PROTEIN**

Heat the oven to 200°C/400°F/gas 6. Peel the peaches by pouring boiling water over them – the skins will loosen within half a minute. If the skins are sound and unblemished, though, don't bother, just wash them very carefully. Halve the fruit, remove the stones, and slice – not too thinly– into a buttered pie dish. Unless the oranges and lemon are unsprayed, scrub the skins meticulously before you grate the rind.

Put the orange and lemon juice in a small pan with the honey and a good powdering of nutmeg, and heat until the honey is melted. Pour half in and around the peaches. Mix the grated orange and lemon rind with the ground almonds, and smooth the mixture over the top. Pour the rest of the juicy sauce over them, put in the oven covered with a piece of foil, and bake for 45 minutes. Greek yogurt makes a luxurious accompaniment to this dish.

| INGREDIENTS |
| --- |
| **4 peaches** |
| **juice and grated rind of 2 oranges** |
| **juice and grated rind of 1 lemon** |
| **3tbs honey** |
| **nutmeg** |
| **50g/2oz ground almonds** |

## BLACKBERRY PARFAIT

### INGREDIENTS

**500g/1lb blackberries**

**2tbs apple juice**

**1tbs clear honey**

**300ml/½pt Greek yogurt**

Wash the blackberries carefully – save a few for decoration. Put the fruit in a pan with the apple juice and honey. Heat over a very low flame until the juices run – a few minutes only – and allow to cool. Then blend or process with the Greek yogurt. Put in a closed, freezer-proof container, and leave in the freezer for a few hours. Take it out and give it a couple of vigorous stirs to break up any crystals that may have formed. Return to the freezer for another 2–3 hours. Just before serving, stir again with a fork, divide between individual glass bowls, and top each serving with yogurt and some blackberries.

PROTEIN

## STEWED APPLES WITH GINGER

### INGREDIENTS

**4–5 crisp eating apples or 3 large Bramleys**

**1tbs apple juice or water**

**2tbs honey**

**2tsp grated fresh ginger**

**1tbs lemon juice**

**grated rind of 1 well-scrubbed lemon**

Peel the apples, and core them. Put them in a big pan with the apple juice or water, the honey, ginger, and lemon juice. Simmer over a low heat until the apples are cooked and fluffy. Take off the heat, turn into a pretty bowl, and scatter the grated lemon rind on top.

PROTEIN

## PEACHES IN WHITE WINE WITH PRESERVED GINGER

### INGREDIENTS

**4 medium peaches**

**about 300ml/½pt chilled white wine – dry, slightly sweet, or sparkling, according to your preference**

**a few pieces of ginger, and 2tbs of the syrup, from a jar or can of preserved ginger**

Skin the peaches. The skins will peel off easily if the peaches are immersed in boiling water for half a minute or even less.

Take 4 wine-glasses and put a peach in each one. Pour over the chilled white wine, put 2 or 3 small pieces of preserved ginger on top, and spoon a little of the strongly flavoured syrup over them.

PROTEIN

# DRIED FRUIT COMPÔTE

**PROTEIN**

Wash the fruit carefully. Boil the water, pour over the rosehip teabag in a china bowl, and leave to steep for 10 minutes. Remove the teabag. Pour the liquid into a pan, add the dried fruit, honey, and cloves, and simmer for 15 minutes. Leave to cool for several hours or overnight. Serve sprinkled with the flaked almonds.

| INGREDIENTS |
| --- |
| 250g/8oz prunes |
| 125g/4oz dried apricots |
| 125g/4oz dried figs |
| 50g/2oz raisins |
| 600ml/1pt water |
| 1 rosehip teabag |
| 2tbs honey |
| 3–4 cloves |
| 25g/1oz flaked almonds, to decorate |

# PUDDINGS FOR STARCH MEALS

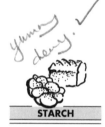

*yummy*
*dear!* ✓

**STARCH**

*Healthier +*
*+*
*hours*

# SPICED RICE CREAM★

Measure the water into a pan, and add the cinnamon sticks, aniseed, cardamon pods, and cloves. Bring to the boil and simmer gently, covered, for 10–15 minutes, until the water has turned brown and absorbed the flavour of the spices.

Strain off the spices (they can be discarded), and make up the water to 300ml/½pt again if it has reduced. Put the well-washed rice in a heavy pan with a lid, and pour the water over it. Add the honey, bring to the boil, then cover. Turn the heat right down, and cook until all the water has been absorbed. Remove the pan from the heat, and let it sit, uncovered, until the rice has dried out a little. (If it is cooked through but still a little wet, pop it in a moderately hot oven to dry out for a couple of minutes.)

When the rice is cold, whip the cream well, and stir it into the rice. Check the flavour, adding a little more honey if necessary. Put the rice mixture in a serving bowl, dust with a sprinkling of powdered nutmeg or cinnamon, and chill until ready to serve.

| INGREDIENTS |
| --- |
| 300ml/½pt water |
| 2 cinnamon sticks |
| 1tsp aniseed |
| 3 cardamon pods |
| 4 whole cloves |
| 175g/6oz short-grain brown rice |
| 2tbs clear honey |
| 150g/5oz double cream |
| cinnamon |
| nutmeg |

## BAKED BANANAS★

### INGREDIENTS

| |
|---|
| 4 bananas |
| 50g/2oz unsalted butter |
| grated nutmeg |
| 2tbs raisins |
| 2tbs sesame seeds |

Heat the oven to 200°C/400°F/gas 6. Peel the bananas, halve them lengthways, and put them side by side in a greased fireproof dish. Dot the butter over them, grate a little nutmeg on top, and sprinkle with the well-washed raisins. Bake for about 10 minutes, turning them over once. Remove them to a clean, warm serving dish, and scatter the toasted sesame seeds on top.

STARCH

## TROPICAL FRUIT SALAD

### INGREDIENTS

| |
|---|
| 125g/4oz sultanas, preferably unsulphured ones |
| 1 cinnamon stick |
| 2–3 cloves |
| 1 ripe mango |
| 2 ripe papayas |
| 2 bananas |
| 2tbs split blanched almonds |

Wash the sultanas and put them in a small pan with a teacupful of water. Add the cinnamon stick and the cloves to the water, and simmer for about half an hour, covered, until the sultanas are soft. Allow the sultanas to cool in their cooking water.

Peel the mango and slice it thinly into a china bowl. Peel the papayas, remove the seeds, and slice into the bowl. Peel and slice the bananas. Strain the cooked sultanas, reserve the cooking water, and discard the spices. Then add to the rest of the fruit. Pour over the sultanas' cooking liquid. Toast the split blanched almonds briefly in a hot frying-pan, and scatter over the fruit.

STARCH

## DRIED FRUIT MINI-BUNS★

### INGREDIENTS

| |
|---|
| 40g/1½oz unsalted butter |
| 125g/4oz wholewheat self-raising flour |
| 1tbs brown sugar |
| 50g/2oz raisins or currants (or both) |
| 1 egg yolk |
| 1tbs milk |

*These useful little buns contain very little sugar. They can be added to a packed lunch, or can fill a teatime gap for those people who are still addicted to sweet foods.*

Heat the oven to 220°C/425°F/gas 7. Crumble the butter into the flour, add the sugar and currants, and mix well. Add the well-beaten egg yolk. At this stage the dough may already be moist enough to come away from the sides of the bowl. If it is not, add the milk. Mix well, and form into 10 or 12 round mini-buns. Put them on a greased baking tin, and bake in the preheated oven for 12–15 minutes or until firm and well-browned.

STARCH

# INDEX